Your Best Golf Begins After 50

Endorsements

"*Your Best Golf Begins After 50* is the perfect read for anyone who dreams of yardage gains and less pains."

Jack Canfield, Coauthor of the #1 *New York Times* bestselling *Chicken Soup for the Soul*® series and *The Success Principles™: How to Get from Where You Are to Where You Want to Be*

"I've spent thousands on golf tools, gimmicks and training with little change to my score card, then I met Barry & Tammy. *Your Best Golf Begins After 50* was the answer for me. If you want to play better golf, start with this book!"

Ken Dunn, author of *WSJ* Bestseller *The Greatest Prospector In The World.*

"Barry and Tammy are masters at what they do. They understand the middle-aged golfer and their needs because they've been there. And now they've put all the key elements of a successful system in one place for you to experience."

Deanna Hansen, author of *Unblock Your Body* and founder of Fluid Isometrics and Block Therapy

"Quite possibly the best husband-and-wife golf combo to ever come out of Manitoba. Tammy and Barry will help you play the best back nine of your life and maybe finish with a few birdies along the way!"

Terry Hashimoto, Manitoba Hall of Fame golfer, golf entrepreneur and researcher, founder of Jazz Golf, BodiTrak, and Swing Balance Solutions

"What makes this book great is the vast knowledge and expertise that Tammy and Barry bring to it, as they've been there. But what really sets it apart from others is their passion for this great game of golf and wanting to help others."

Rob McMillan, Professional Golfer,
three-time Canadian PGA Tour Winner

"If you only read one golf book this year, this is the one you need to have in your hands!"

Patty Aubery, Coauthor of the #1 *New York Times* bestselling *Chicken Soup for the Soul*® series former president of Jack Canfield Companies

"Having worked extensively in elite sport for the past twenty-seven years, I can attest that this is easily the best book on golf performance I've had the pleasure to read. Tammy and Barry bring their tremendous experience and expertise throughout the book and position the ideas on the body-swing connection while acknowledging the importance of the holistic aspects to one's overall golf performance. Regardless of our age, we can always find opportunities for improvement and growth, and this book will guide the reader along a path of playing their best golf into their fifties and beyond."

Dr Tom Patrick, PhD
Sydney, Australia

"I began working on the game of golf later in life as it provides a breadth and depth of life-long learning that transcends sport and provides a meaningful metaphor for living! Tammy and Barry provide the perfect balance of the triangle of swing, physical training and mental training needed in game improvement and more important—game enjoyment! The ideas in their book are life changing!"

Karen Yamada, aspiring senior golfer
Winnipeg, Manitoba, Canada

—YOUR— Best Golf Begins After 50

Make the Back Nine Your Best Nine

TAMMY AND BARRY GIBSON

NEW YORK

LONDON • NASHVILLE • MELBOURNE • VANCOUVER

Your Best Golf Begins After 50

Make Your Back Nine Your Best Nine

Published in New York, New York, by Morgan James Publishing. Morgan James is a trademark of Morgan James, LLC. www.MorganJamesPublishing.com

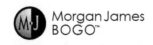

ISBN 9781631954320 paperback
ISBN 9781631954337 eBook
Library of Congress Control Number: 2020950673

Cover and Interior Design by:
Chris Treccani
www.3dogcreative.net

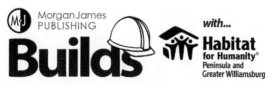

Morgan James is a proud partner of Habitat for Humanity Peninsula and Greater Williamsburg. Partners in building since 2006.

Get involved today! Visit
MorganJamesPublishing.com/giving-back

Contents

Acknowledgments

Writing this book was truly a labor of love for both of us and more rewarding than we could ever have imagined.

We would like to first give a special thanks to our daughter, Kelsey, who put up with all our crazy business shenanigans, always supporting and encouraging us even though she really wasn't sure what we were doing.

Thanks to Jack Canfield, whose guidance and mentoring first led us down this path of taking responsibility for our lives and believing anything is possible. We will be forever grateful!

Thanks to Deanna Hansen, who introduced us to the world of fascia health, Block Therapy and helped us begin our journey of restoring our health, our vitality, and our golf.

Thanks to Ken Dunn and Nicolas Boothman for introducing us to their Writing Madly Weekend that helped us to bring this book out of our heads and into the world.

Thanks to David Hancock and everyone on the Morgan James Publishing team who helped us to make this book a reality and contributed to our success.

Thanks to our students, whose constant faith in us pushed us harder to be better for them.

And thanks to the universe for bringing the right people to us at the right time to make this book and our journey together happen.

We are forever grateful to this great game of golf which has been woven through our lives, providing us with so many amazing experiences and being a big catalyst for helping us live a healthier, happier life. Our journey is to give back and share this wonderful experience and great game with others.

Introduction

Golf is the closest game to the game we call life. You get bad breaks from good shots; you get good breaks from bad shots—but you have to play the ball where it lies.
–Bobby Jones, Golf Great

Aging is inevitable and this book is not about avoiding it, but rather embracing it to play your best golf ever. It's not accepting the status quo of "I'm getting older" and instead believing the "back nine can indeed be your best nine". That's what this great game of golf has taught us in our journey, and we want to share it with you. Having the attitude of "forever young" is a great positive mindset, but we also want to live and move in a body that's forever young, maintaining our mobility, flexibility, and our health so we can play the best golf of our life in the back nine of life.

What if you could have a simple and easy way to help you play the best golf of your life, well into your fifties and beyond, and help you stay fit and healthy doing it? Would you be interested? Many golfers just accept that their golf will get worse as they age! Our life expectancy as humans has increased over time and we are now living longer, and some of us healthier. But for many people as they age, they accept weight gains, declining energy levels, loss of mobility, loss of strength, increased aches and pains and other related health issues as normal. More than 80 percent of golfers over the age of fifty have back pain or other mobility issues when they play golf. And because of this they can't play golf to the best of their ability or enjoy the game and life to the fullest. That *was* us.

We are lovers of life and golf. Our mission is to inspire and motivate golfers all over the world to play the best golf of their lives and to get healthier doing it. Tammy is a competitive amateur golfer, competing for over thirty years, and Barry is a PGA of Canada golf professional for thirty-plus years. Both of us have overcome major health issues in our fifties and are now playing the best golf of our lives. We were motivated to write this book because we want you to play the best golf of your life too!

Barry was a scratch golfer for most of his life until his thirties, but his passion is teaching others. The long days on his feet resulted in back problems, and for twenty years he lived with constant pain. He also started adding on the pounds by turning to comfort food. Daily living was a struggle. Tammy was dealing with high stress levels in her office job, and over the years she developed chronic neck and shoulder pain due to poor posture, compounded by progressive hip pain. Arthritis in the hip joints ran rampant in her family.

Over the years, both of us tried many therapies and techniques, and some worked to varying degrees, but they only gave us limited, short-term relief. Then we discovered a new and innovative technique that changed all that. After three months of practicing this technique, Barry's back was 75 percent better and Tammy's hip pain was gone. After nine months, Barry was moving and lifting heavy furniture with no pain at all in his back. Tammy's chronic neck and shoulder pain disappeared. Both of us started playing the best golf of our lives. Tammy is now a five-time provincial amateur champion, and Barry is a top golf teaching professional. We have since helped hundreds of our students feel better, move better, and play better, on and off the golf course.

Our years of research and knowledge empowered us to create this unique system that has brought health back to our bodies, success back to our golf game, and more fun and joy into our lives. We know what it's like not to be able to play your best golf. We've been there. But we found a way to change all that. And as we move into the "back nine" of our lives, we want it to be the best nine. We want that for you too. We want to share our success formula with you so you can have that experience as well and play the best golf of your life.

Who This Book Is For

This book differs from other golf books because we focus specifically on you, the fifty-plus golfer, and give you a simple and easy approach that integrates body health, mindset, and golf technique into one whole system that will make you feel better, move better, and play better, on and off the course. This will allow you to play the game you are so passionate about for as long as you like.

Maybe you are suffering with back pain, joint pain, mobility issues, and even limiting beliefs about how you can keep playing as you age. You really love the game but are wondering whether or not you should keep playing if you can't enjoy it anymore. You are looking for answers.

Wouldn't you like to experience playing the best golf of your life into your seventies, eighties, even nineties? Read on, this is for you!

What's Coming Up

In the pages ahead we'll explore what it is that draws us to this awesome game and why it's so important for us all to keep playing our best as we age. We'll talk about taking stock of your current situation and circumstances regarding your game. What are the challenges you're facing right now to play your best? How long has it been that way? What have you done to change it?

We'll explain how you can create a vision for your "back nine" and set realistic and achievable goals for that vision. We'll discuss ways to take action on those goals and keep them manageable. Throughout the book each of us will share stories that further illustrate a topic or simply make our golf journeys more "real" to you as the reader. Those sections will be set off with our names in boldface, like the subtitle you see above. So whenever you see **Tammy's Story** or **Barry's Story**, just know that an anecdote will follow.

We'll also talk about the golf swing and the basic components of a good swing. Then we'll present some common swing faults that people over fifty have and why they have them. We'll give you solutions and drills to correct those faults and help you stay motivated to keep moving forward.

We'll present some very unique mind-body connection techniques we use that are like having a "superpower" for playing great golf.

And finally, we'll help you pull this all together so that you can keep playing your best golf today and every day.

Our promise to you is that if you follow our system, you'll play better golf, have better mobility, play with less pain, and have more fun. You'll be able to enjoy your golf and life to the fullest. We'll keep this promise by offering you continuing support through our online community, if you choose to join us.

You can always play better and be better, no matter your age. Make the back nine bogey-free. Make it your best nine.

Chapter 1:

A Good Walk Ruined

Most of us golfers are fanatics. We love the game! Why is that? What draws us to this intriguing and mind-wracking game? Many people who have never golfed don't quite get why golfers are addicted to the game. Or if they've played once or twice, they found it so frustrating that they quit right then. Non-golfers just don't get the lure of the game.

Tammy's Story

I remember the first time I walked down a fairway playing my first round of golf. It was a rural nine-hole course where you just showed up, put your $10 green fee in an envelope, and slipped it into a small wooden lockbox. Okay, I know I'm dating myself, but that was how it went down. There was a lot of trust

1

back then! My golfing partner, Phyllis, was excited to have someone to play with as very few other women played golf at this course.

Phyllis and I had met through work, and she asked if I golfed. (I had always wanted to golf but never had.) I blurted out, "Yeah, of course I golf. I love it." Why I said that I don't know. I think I must have imagined golfing in my head so much I truly felt I could, and so it just came out of my mouth. I borrowed an old set of my uncle's clubs and got ready to play my first game.

So there we were walking down the first fairway, and I had to live up to my declaration that I knew how to play golf. I had played baseball for years so figured if I could swing at a moving ball and hit it, I could easily make contact with a little white ball sitting on a little wooden tee!

Thankfully, I made contact with the ball on my first tee shot, keeping it in the fairway but not very far, maybe 150 yards. The next shots would be telltale. I remember not even thinking anything of it. I just knew I would be able to hit the ball okay and scrape my way around the course as if I knew what I was doing. Golf seemed natural for me and it was something that excited me, revved me up. I think I loved the game before I actually played it.

Those of you who love the game know this feeling. The game calls to us. If you ask golfers, you will get a multitude of reasons why they golf, but we think it all comes down to a few common ones. We'd like to share them with you.

Good for Your Health

This a biggie, and we know it firsthand. Golfing isn't just good for your health; it's *great* for your health. This is why playing golf into your fifties and later can be so good for you; it will actually make you heathier. Do you know that each time you walk an 18 hole golf course, you are walking approximately five miles? Think of all the great exercise and fresh air you are getting. You can burn up to 1400 calories when you walk eighteen holes (and even as many as 800 when you ride a power cart!). Walking is very good for the heart, and it helps with your breathing as well, if you're mindful of *how* you are breathing. We'll talk more about breathing later.

Being outdoors in nature has a calming effect on the body. When you play golf you are in the moment. You can appreciate and be grateful for what you see around you. Even if you are not golfing, being in nature on its own has great health benefits. There is a connection with nature that occurs because we are part of it.

Believe it or not, golfing can reduce stress. That's because as you exercise your body releases endorphins, the feel-good hormone. As you start to feel better, the worries and stresses of the day fade away. Although you may have some stress about your golf shot, your other stresses in life are gone for this moment in time as you focus on your game.

A review in the *British Journal of Sports Medicine* in 2016 concluded that golf "improved physical health and mental well-being, and is a potential contribution to increased life expectancy."[1] Another study published by the same journal in 2018 found that "golf is associated with increased life expectancy, improved cardiovascular risk factors, and mental well-being."[2] So, you see, golfing really is good for your health.

A Nineteen Hole Game

Golf is the ultimate sport for socializing. It's a great way to meet new people and make new friends. Over the years, we have met so many amazing people in our golf travels and made lifelong friends. And as we get older, it's important for us to keep up our social connections as it contributes to better mental health in old age.

Typically, when you play golf, you are playing with your friends or clubmates. You're enjoying walking down the fairway, catching up on news, sharing stories, and maybe even discussing your golf shots. Afterwards, at the nineteenth hole, you might enjoy some refreshments and rehash all your shots and comical events that happened during the round. All this social connection is important

---

1 "The relationships between golf and health: a scoping review," Murray et al, *British Journal of Sports Medicine*, https://bjsm.bmj.com/content/51/1/12

2 "2018 International Consensus Statement on Golf and Health to guide action by people, policymakers and the golf industry," *British Journal of Sports Medicine*, Murray et al, https://bjsm.bmj.com/content/52/22/1426.long

for your health. Your brain is wired to connect and interact with others, it's at the core of your physical and mental health.

Golfing gets you interacting with like-minded people. These positive social interactions improve your quality of life, boost your mental health, and help you live longer. Being socially connected as we age is more important than ever in our increasingly isolated world.

And then there is the fun factor. For us, this is one of the most important reasons we like to play golf—it brings us a lot of joy! Golf can bring out a lot of emotions when you play, almost every emotion you experience in life. But experiencing joy, having fun, and being able to laugh at yourself are the best feelings of all.

Barry's Story

We were on the sixteenth hole at our club. One of the guys in our foursome, Dean, hit his second shot into the pond along the left fairway. The ball was half in and half out of the water by the rocks. Being a true golfer to the core, and not wanting to take a penalty stroke, he took off his socks and shoes and stood almost up to his knees in water so he could take a swing at the half-submerged golf ball. *Swack!* The ball came sailing out of the water hazard and landed on the green. Dean ... well, he wasn't so lucky. He lost his balance and fell backward into the water, getting soaked from head to toe! The rest of us were hysterical with laughter. Dean was okay; only his pride was hurt. He laughed at himself as he sloshed his way out of the water hazard. We chuckled the rest of the way around the course with that image in our heads, and we also played our best golf! Laughter really *is* great for your game and for your health.

Challenge Yourself

Although golf is a social game played with others, it's an individual sport as well. It's a game you can play by yourself and against yourself. Even if you are in a group, you are always challenging yourself individually. It's you against the course. It's you against yourself. You are always growing and learning. And that's essential for keeping your brain healthy and your game improving as you get older.

If you are competitive in nature, this is a great sport to challenge yourself each time you're out playing. Competing brings out a drive in some people that really excites them. The thing is, perfection in golf is elusive—and that's what keeps us coming back. But if you work hard at it you can get great results. Many people love this type of challenge and love to compete.

Tammy has competed at sports all throughout her life. In golf, she's played in club competitions, provincial championships, and national championships. The competition aspect drives her. And this is what drives many other people as well. Competing helped her learn about how to strategize, plan, set goals, and take action around her love for the game. This all led her to become a five-time provincial amateur champion.

For others, competition may mean playing at a club event or just competing against your foursome in a snips game, or even against yourself. You're trying to better yourself, trying to better your own score each time. Whatever the motivation, it's something that is going to work just for you. It will meet whatever your needs are for competition.

The unique and appealing thing about golf is that you can never be perfect at it. But you can keep trying to do the best you can. This is how life is as well. Golf imitates life. It helps you to keep moving forward, continually challenging yourself to be better.

We want a win-win situation. That's the best scenario. When you're trying to win, when you're trying to improve at golf, you are improving at life as well. Just keep at it and don't give up. Golf is the closest thing to the game we call life. It can be a good walk ruined, or it can be a great walk made even better. That's up to you. There is so much this game can teach us about our lives, about ourselves, and about others. You can derive much joy and wonderful experiences and memories from golf.

This book was written during the height of the coronavirus pandemic in the summer and fall of 2020, and when other sport and fitness activities were restricted, golf was one of the few sports allowed to stay open. The health benefits were recognized. And because golf is played outdoors on many acres of land, social distancing and other safety and health protocols were easy to put in place. The game allowed people to get outdoors and enjoy nature, and to socialize and connect with others. It also encouraged people to get some exercise and feel alive again. Golf really was a lifesaver for some.

So however you slice it—or hook it or fade it or draw it—golf certainly is a way to get a "hole-in-one" in the game of healthy long living.

Chapter 2:

Bogies or Birdies

Where are you right now with your golf game? What you are doing, or not doing, may be hindering your golf game and your ability to play your best. Let's do an assessment and see.

Play and Practice

How often do you play golf right now? How often do you practice? Do you even like to practice? Why or why not?

Many people when they arrive at the course just head straight out to the first tee to play. No warm-up, no hitting balls, no stretching. Just off to the first tee. *Swack!* Straight down the middle … or not. If you practice, how often? Three times a week? Once a week? Do a quick mental assessment of this and then jot it down. Having a baseline for your play and practice time will help you determine what else is needed to get you from where you are to where you want to be in your golf game.

When Tammy first started competing, she knew instinctively that a lot of practice was critical for her to improve her game.

"I was the type of player that needed to practice more than I played. I would schedule three or more practice sessions a week and work hard to make that happen. No excuses if I wanted to improve my game."

Do you have a weekly or monthly routine of play, or is it haphazard? Why is that? As we mentioned above, knowing how much you play on a weekly or monthly basis will help you determine what you need to do to achieve your golfing goals. Do you take lessons? Why or why not? Some people take lessons for years and never improve. Yet others take a few lessons and improve dramatically right away. Where are you in this scenario? Why have lessons either worked or not worked for you in the past? Have you practiced between your lessons?

Remember, you must do the work. Doing this initial assessment of where you are *right now* will give you the foundational information you need to move forward.

Fitness and Wellbeing

Let's talk about mobility issues and chronic pain when you golf. This is something we know a lot about, having dealt with it ourselves for the past twenty years. These are two key reasons why many golfers play less golf after fifty—the inability to move properly in the golf swing and suffering with aches and pain during and after a round. These can be debilitating for many golfers.

Your level of health and fitness is a key factor that will determine your ability to enjoy this great game. A great deal of body movement and coordination is required in golf, and if your body is in pain or you can't move well when you play … that's no fun. As you get older the key is to keep moving every day, at least thirty minutes a day if you can. If you are not staying mobile, fit, and flexible, you run the risk of developing pain and disease that will inhibit your ability to enjoy your golf game and, for that matter, your life.

We talked earlier about how golf provides a form of exercise. But what about exercise outside of golf? Do you do any? If so, what? We can't stress enough how important it is to keep moving every day as you age, otherwise you will begin to experience mobility issues in your golf and your daily functional health.

When doing workouts, it's healthier for your body as you age to do more dynamic stretching than weightlifting. Dynamic stretching will give you greater movement in your joints and improves your posture. It also helps to release muscle tension and pain or soreness, and reduces the risk of injury. Dynamic stretching may also help increase your circulation, strengthen muscle control, and improve your balance and coordination. All these are necessary for peak performance in golf and maintaining a healthy body. We all want to practice active aging. The secret is to stretch and be active when you are younger. This will benefit you immensely as you age.

"You are what you eat." Have you heard that before? What you put in your body will fuel you for golf. If you put in junk food, that's poor fuel. If you put in nutritious foods, that's powerful fuel. Do you know if you're getting the right nutrients every day to fuel you up? How about during a round of golf? Do you have snacks? What do you eat and drink? Many of us don't realize how much of an impact this has on our golf performance.

Over the past ten years we have slowly switched from a heavy red meat diet to a more plant-based diet and cut out as much sugar as we could. We also eliminated all diet soft drinks and other sugary beverages. As a result of these changes, we both lost those few extra pounds that were creeping on, we feel better, we move better, and we have a ton more energy. Don't get us wrong, we still like a good steak once in a while, but we now eat a lot more vegetables, chicken and fish. We are not nutritional experts, but we have educated ourselves over the years and have enough personal experience to know what works best for us. We use a common-sense approach. We raise the topic of nutrition here so you will remember to pay attention to it going forward; it's another important factor affecting your health and your golf performance. There is plenty of good information available elsewhere on this topic, so do your homework and see what works best for you.

Playing while in pain is another factor to be assessed. When you play, do you experience pain? If so, in what areas of your body? How long have you had the pain? Does it go away after you play? Are you seeing a medical doctor about any of these issues? All of these questions need to be assessed before you can determine your plan to move forward from where you are to where you want to be.

Now let's talk about work-life balance. Are you working full-time right now and trying to fit golf in? Are you retired and playing golf every day? There is a balance we need to strive for and everyone will be different. What works for one will not work for others. It all comes back to deciding what you want out of your golf. Shoot lower scores? Hit it farther? Become more competitive? Play with less pain? Once you know this, you can devise a plan that will fit you.

Tammy's Story

When I was in my teens, I recall many of my older relatives complained of aches and pains and other health issues. They had difficulty climbing stairs and very easily got out of breath. Many were overweight. They all had arthritis in their joints, and all eventually needed hip and knee replacements.

My mom has had both hips replaced *twice*, one knee replaced *twice*, and six screws put in her left ankle, all because of arthritis.

I thought, *Oh no, I'm destined to this same fate! Arthritis runs in my family, and I won't be able to escape it.* I knew I did not want to end up with this crippling disease as an adult but thought I had no choice. I then made a decision in my early twenties to educate myself on causes of arthritis and learned that if I stayed fit and active, and at a healthy weight, I might be able to at least prolong the onset of arthritis and enjoy normal mobility for a long time into old age. I believed I had a choice about my health! This belief motivated me and I became very active in many sports, I quit smoking (yes, I was a smoker in my teens—stupid, huh?), and paid more attention to what I ate and drank. In my twenties and thirties, I was very healthy and active, and into fitness.

And as I continued to play more golf, being fit helped me to become more competitive with absolutely no arthritis anywhere and no medication needed for pain. However, as I aged and moved into my early fifties, I became lazy and the weight packed on and aches and pains started to appear, and increase! The adage "you're just getting old, accept it" crept into my thoughts and I believed it … for a while. But then I remembered, I had a choice about my health and I was able to tackle it head on and win my health back.

I attribute that win, in part, to a new and extraordinary self-care fascia release practice we discovered, a practice that I am now trained in to teach others. I am convinced this ground-breaking technique has helped to keep arthritis and any other joint issues at bay as I age because of its unique healing abilities. You'll hear more about this in Chapter 6. My message here is that you must stay active, eat well, and keep your weight in control if you want to avoid chronic pain and disease as you age. You may play some of your best golf then! I did.

What Have You Tried?

Barry had years of back pain and mobility issues in his thirties and early forties. Much of it was from a lifetime of traumas, old sports injuries, lifestyle, and general golf repetitive motion strain, which culminated in the classic lumbar L5-S1 disk herniation his back, very common for golfers. The frustrating part for him was that no one could really solve or explain the pain. He tried many therapies and medications over the years that helped to a degree, but they were never long-lasting—until he started using the new self-care fascia release technique mentioned above. He now feels great and is relatively pain-free!

How about you? How do you feel? Are you on medication to help you deal with existing health conditions or chronic pain? Do these medications help you when you golf, or do they hinder you? When we were on medications and pain relievers, we found that some helped ease the pain, but they also made us "loopy" or drowsy, resulting in poor balance and depth perception. Have you asked yourself if all these medications are really necessary? We are by no means saying you should go off any medication but rather suggesting that you may need to reassess why you need them.

What about physical therapy treatments? Many people in their fifties and older seek out chiropractors, massage therapists, or physiotherapists to help relieve their pain. These therapies do provide relief, but unless you are doing some type of ongoing self-care in between you'll need to keep going for treatments. And for some people that can get very expensive, so they quit going.

How often do you go for treatments? What do you do between treatment sessions? Do you do yoga or Pilates or other modalities that can help you? Maybe you haven't tried anything? We would find that hard to believe, because if you're reading this book, we know you're the type of person who wants to look after your health so you can play better golf. You are likely doing physical activities to help your game without even realizing it. You may not consciously connect that a walk in the evening may help you play better golf. Or doing yoga or breathing practice. Or walking the dog. Or playing with the grandkids in the park. There are many other activities you could be doing. Assess everything you are doing so you have a good baseline of data going forward.

Chapter 3:

Focus on the Target and Follow-Through

Okay, so you've assessed why you golf and where you are at. Now let's talk about what you want. What do you really want out of your golf game? Do you want to shoot lower scores? Do you want to hit the ball farther? Do you want to be a better putter? Do you want to be a better bunker player? Maybe you want to play more often or practice more. Maybe you just want to play without aches and pains. Whatever it is, you need to decide and be clear on what you want. If you don't know what you want, how will you know when you get it?

Decide What You Want

Many people don't get what they want because they haven't *actually* decided what they want. They haven't described their desires in clear and convincing detail, or they are not willing to accept responsibility for what they want.

So let's go back to that question. What do you want to accomplish in your golf game? What do you want to experience on (and off) the golf course? What skill level do you want to achieve— weekend warrior, competitive amateur, successful tour player? What does success in your golf look like to you?

- Hitting the ball straighter and farther?
- Shooting lower scores?
- Becoming a better putter?
- Playing a round pain-free?
- Having a better mindset so you can get in the "zone" and stay there?
- Becoming a club, provincial/state, national champion?
- Achieving a better work-life balance?
- Maybe all of these things?

You *must* decide this and be very clear and specific about what you want. But having said that, it also means you are responsible to do the work.

And when asked a question, you need to stop saying "I don't know," "I don't care," or "It doesn't matter to me." When faced with a choice, no matter how small or insignificant, act as if you care, as if you have a preference, and make a choice about what you want.

Once you are clear and focused on *what* you want, *how* you'll get it will show up. This happens through something in your brain called the reticular activating system or RAS.

The RAS is a complex network of neurons and connective pathways in your brain that connects to the spinal cord and body. The RAS takes what you focus on and creates a filter for it. It then filters the data coming in and brings to your attention only those things important to you. This happens at a subconscious level without you even noticing. Pretty awesome, right?

Let's look at an example. If you believe you are poor at putting, you probably will be because you are always sending that negative data to your brain through your thoughts. If you believe you are a great driver of the ball, you most likely are. Your RAS helps you see what you want to see and in doing so influences your actions.

So here's the magic! You can train your RAS by aligning your subconscious thoughts with your conscious thoughts. This is called "setting your intent." It basically means that if you focus hard on what you want, your RAS will reveal the people, information, and opportunities that will help you get what you want. If you really want to improve your golf game, set your intention and you'll tune in to the right information and actions that help you achieve it. Focus on negative thoughts and you will invite negativity into your life. Focus on positive things and they will come to you because your brain is seeking them out. You have that choice. It's like having a superpower!

To train your RAS, create a vision in your mind of what you want and then let your subconscious and conscious minds work together to make it happen. Write your vision down and keep it close at hand. Read and reread it often. This will continually refocus and remind your brain about what matters and what doesn't. It moves you toward your goals—toward what you want.

A good example of using this visioning technique is Rory McIlroy. McIlroy decided at a very young age he would be the best golfer in the world. He had a vision for what he wanted and was very clear about it. He continually kept his vision top of mind as he grew older. He stated it publicly whenever he had the opportunity so that made him accountable. His RAS was programmed to seek those things that would give him the outcomes he wanted. And, as they say, the rest is history.

Some of the areas we both focus on in our visioning process are listed below. Use these as a guide to help you come up with your own.

- Increased strength for power to hit the ball farther.
- Consistently shooting lower scores.
- Less pain in back and joints.
- Greater flexibility and mobility for ease of swing.
- Better mental focus for clarity and concentration, getting in the "zone".
- Overcoming fears or nervousness on the first tee.

- Playing in tournaments and competitions—and winning!

Think about how these aspects of your vision are affecting you on and off the golf course. Ask yourself: How do I look and feel in that future state when I have achieved my vision in each area? Creating the feelings around your vision is critical. It's what helps create your new positive memory for that area.

Set a time frame for achieving your vision. For example, a year from now, what would you like to have happened in each area? Try to come up with one or two things for each area. Write it down; this makes it real. Then share your vision with a friend, partner, family member, or your trainer—it holds you accountable. Remember to read your vision every day. The best times are when you first wake up and before you go to bed. Repeating this will continually refocus and remind your brain about what you want. You are reprogramming your RAS.

One of our clients, Karen, plays golf almost six times a week. She came to us with a very clear vision for what she wanted: more flexibility in her core, greater speed through the ball, more power. She knew exactly what she wanted; she was very specific. Her goals then could be focused on her vision, and she would not get drawn into wasting time on other things. The amazing thing was that by focusing on the things she wanted she also received side benefits of getting more distance and losing a bit of weight, which were things she wanted to eventually address. Her RAS brought her more of what she wanted.

Let's summarize what you've learned here. First, you need to be very clear in your mind about what you want. Then you need to write it down. Once you've written it down, imagine already having it. What does it look like, feel like, sound like, smell like, taste like? Use all your senses. Do this for each area you want to change. Be very clear on it. Once you have your visions cemented in your brain, it will be so much easier to set goals around these areas.

Focus on the Target

The next step in your journey is to set goals based on your vision. To help ensure you achieve your goals, you want them to be SMART. This means they need to be Specific, Measurable, Achievable, Realistic, and Time-bound.

For example, instead of setting a goal "To play better golf", make it SMART and say, "To be scoring in the 70s for eighty percent of my rounds played, by December 31, 2021". Or instead of setting a goal "To play golf more often", your SMART goal might be "To play golf every Monday, Wednesday and Friday morning during May to September." If you aren't specific about your goals, you have less chance to achieve them.

Tammy's Story

When I was in my late twenties, my vision was to be a top-caliber golfer. I set a goal to be a provincial team member and represent my province in golf. Always competitive by nature, I instinctively knew that to get what I wanted I had to set goals. Playing on the provincial team was what I wanted. My SMART goal was "To become a member of the Manitoba provincial amateur women's golf team by the age of thirty-five." I was a late bloomer on the competitive scene and had to contend with all the young twenty year olds. So how was I going to achieve this big goal? The first thing I did was create a series of process goals to help me get there. These were:

- Play a minimum of three times a week during the golf season.
- Practice four times a week during the golf season.
- Play with better golfers during seventy-five percent of rounds played.
- Do exercise and strength training program three times a week during the off season.
- Follow a specific nutrition plan for off season and golf season.
- Work with a sports psychologist and practice mindset training five days a week both in off season and golf season.

So I did all of this. It was a bit overwhelming at first, but I broke it down into smaller chunks, smaller actions, based on priorities. I had to decide what my priorities would be during the golf season and what was better to do in the off season. That made it much more manageable and not so overwhelming for me.

To accelerate achievement of my goals I practiced the visualization technique. The concept here is to rehearse seeing in your mind what you want to happen in reality.

I practiced visualization the entire winter and spring leading up to my provincial championship event in the summer of 1998, where I would try to qualify for the top four spots to make the team. I visualized playing the championship round hole by hole —each swing, each putt—hitting perfect shots each time. I was sinking all those 6- to 8-foot putts for birdies. I was in the zone, nothing could distract me. I could see, feel, hear, touch, and smell victory. It was a fifty-four-hole championship (three rounds), and I would play a round in my head each night, the same way every time. After I got through the third round, I would visualize myself scoring within the top four, being announced as a team member, and accepting my award.

What *actually* happened ended up a bit different. I was in third place after round one and in second place after round two, a few shots behind the leader. During the third round I stuck to my routine as I had visualized. I was really in the zone and didn't even know my score; I just knew I was playing "very steady." On the eighteenth hole, I hit the green in regulation and made a nice two-putt for par. After shaking hands with my competitors, I signed my scorecard and handed it in. The scorer was my friend Carol. She checked the scorecard over, added it up again, and then looked at me with a grin and said, "Well, that settles it. You are number one."

I said, "Excuse me!"

"You are number one," she repeated. "You won!" Until that time I had not been nervous at all. I was just playing out my vision to finish in the top four to make the team. I didn't expect to be number one! I hadn't played that scenario out in my mind, and all of a sudden I became very nervous. I was trembling as she shook my hand and then gave me a big hug to congratulate me. I had not only achieved my goal of making the provincial team, I also won the event. I was the 1998 provincial women's amateur champion! How good is that? Whenever I think back on this story, I always smile. Remember, stay focussed on your target by setting goals and visualizing them becoming a reality. It works. It really does!

Follow-Through

At this point in your journey you should know what you want and have set some goals around that. A great start. You're on your way!

But wait. Right now these are just thoughts in your head and words on paper. How will you make them happen? The answer is you need to follow through by taking action. Taking action is the key to all success. If you don't take action, nothing will change, no matter how much you wish it to be so.

Taking action can be hard for many people. Some of you may feel overwhelmed with all that needs to be done to keep yourself moving forward. Here's our secret sauce to make this work: chunk it down into small pieces. This will make it much more doable, and you'll have much greater success. Pick two or three things that are top priority for you and deal with them first. Perhaps some things may be better dealt with in the offseason—defer those till that time. Once your goal is chunked down you can do it one piece at a time.

Another technique we use to keep us motivated to take action is the "rule of five.", which we learned from our mentor Jack Canfield. The idea here is to pick five small actions or tasks you will commit to doing each day that will move you closer to your goal. Write those five tasks down, either the night before or first thing in the morning of the day you are doing them. Then, to make this more effective, share your task list with a friend, family member, or coach so you are accountable for achieving them. If you don't get everything on your list done that day, carry the unachieved task over to the next day. But try not to carry any tasks over for more than three days. If you do, you may need to rethink whether that is a task you should be doing at this time.

The overall message here is to take some level of action every day that will move you closer to your goal. It doesn't matter how small. It could be making a phone call to book a golf lesson you've been putting off. Or starting a morning walk as part of your exercise routine. Anything that moves you closer to your goal, as long as you take action.

Chapter 4:

The Golf Swing: Common Faults and Fixes

Now we're ready to delve into the golf swing. In this chapter we'll discuss the fundamentals of the golf swing and what makes a "good" golf swing. We'll also present some of the common swing faults we see in a lot of middle-aged golfers and give you some simple and easy fixes. So let's get started.

The Golf Swing

The golf swing is a rotational movement pattern based on body rotation, particularly the separation between the upper and lower body and how the pelvis moves and upper body pivots. These movements are central to the entire golf swing.

Good players rotate and pivot very well and have great separation between the upper and lower body. They can easily and effectively rotate the upper and lower body independently of one another. Some people think this ability is based solely upon good technique. It's true that good players are very athletic and have a high level of coordination. But they also have tremendous hip mobility and excellent upper body (thoracic) mobility, which allows them to turn more easily and effectively. Hence, this leads to good golf technique.

If you've watched players on the PGA and LPGA tours, you've no doubt noticed the various body types and different ways to swing the golf club. For some, the club goes back far and long on the backswing, some have a short backswing, some have fast swings, some have slower swings, some are upright swings, some are flat, some look awkward, and some are flowing and beautiful to look at. But they all work effectively, and these golfers all play to a very high level. The reason for this is all these players have the ability to move and rotate their bodies consistently and efficiently to generate speed, power, and accuracy in their golf games.

Measurement of a golfer's movement pattern is called the "kinematic sequence". It describes the sequence of motion of the body and the golf club—it's like the fingerprint of the swing. All top-level players, regardless of how their swing looks, have a common efficient movement pattern, or a common kinematic sequence.

What does this mean to the average golfer, and how does it help improve your mobility and movement patterns? The kinematic sequence gives you an understanding of the overall required movement patterns for a better swing motion. It allows you to look at your swing, not so much to see what's wrong with it or how it looks, but rather to show how and where you can move more efficiently to make your swing better.

For example, the general movement pattern for good players on the backswing is a centered body pivot around a fixed axis, your spine, whereby the clubhead moves first to start the backswing, followed by the lead arm, the torso, and then the hips and lower body.

On the downswing through striking the golf ball, that body motion reverses. The lower body starts first with the feet and ankles, then the hips and torso, the lead arm, and finally the clubhead. The clubhead is the last to move on the downswing. This results in the efficient, consistent development of power and accuracy.

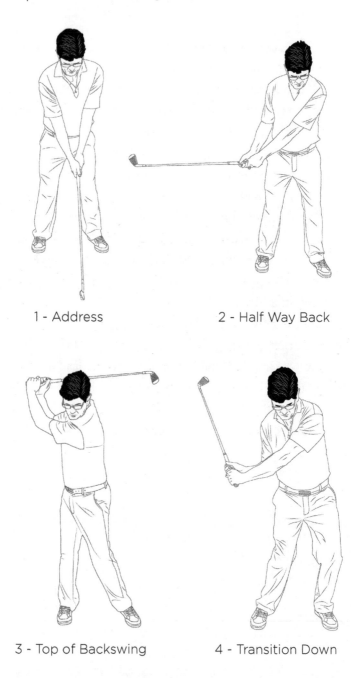

1 - Address

2 - Half Way Back

3 - Top of Backswing

4 - Transition Down

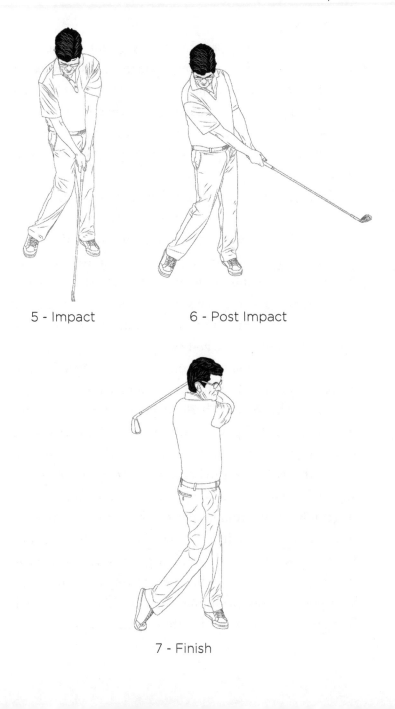

5 - Impact

6 - Post Impact

7 - Finish

With this swing pattern, each segment of the body moves in the correct sequence, which builds and generates speed to the next segment and finally to the clubhead. Hence you end up with maximum acceleration and speed through the striking of the golf ball. This is the same pattern of motion for all good swings despite how the swing may look.

What we are telling you is there is no one best way to swing a golf club. There are many, many ways to swing a club, but there's really only one efficient way for your body to move to generate speed, power, and consistency. The inherent pattern of motion for good swings is the same no matter how the swing looks. This ties into the concept of the body swing connection and the importance of mobility and flexibility in the golf swing.

As you age, you may notice that your body doesn't move as efficiently as it used to. You may find that it gets harder to take the club back properly. Your body doesn't unwind through the ball as well as it once did. The swing gets out of sequence, you lose posture. The chain of motion in the swing starts to breakdown. Then you get inconsistent. The swing is just not going to repeat. You also start to get injuries as a result. Now you have general aches and pains. You attribute it to old age, but actually it's caused by faulty movement patterns. The good news is this can all be reversed, it can all be changed. Starting with improving your posture, your breathing, and your mobility, you will begin to feel better, get rid of those aches and pains, and at the same time play better golf. We'll tell you how you can do all that, but first let's talk about swing faults.

Common Swing Faults

The most common swing faults we see in middle-aged and older golfers are the dreaded slice, the hook, lack of power, and inconsistent contact. Below are scenarios we see all the time. Maybe you can relate?

Brenda, an avid golfer, was on the tee, driver in hand, ready to hit her first shot. *Whack.* "There's my banana slice again, into the trees," she said. Brenda has been playing for twenty years and is now fifty-five. She still has that same bad swing fault. She has tried lesson after lesson to get rid of it, but nothing worked. Why is that? Why does someone suffer so long with a swing fault they can't fix?

Then there's Bob, fifty years old, six-foot-four and 250 pounds of muscle. Bob was as strong as an ox but couldn't hit his driver over 200 yards. What's up with that?

And finally there's Mark, fifty-seven years old. He is average to small build, kind of a wiry guy, and has a great looking golf swing, but there's no power behind it. He could sometimes hit it around 230 yards, but has no consistency or sustained power. He is always exhausted by the thirteenth hole and has no more energy. Why are these players struggling with these issues in their fifties?

We'll say it again. Slicing, hooking, lack of power, and inconsistent play are the major swing faults of all golfers over fifty. Many of these swing faults can be attributed to body movement patterns rather than being a swing fault, per se. Golfers usually think there is something wrong with their swing—"I have to fix my swing"—rather than looking at the movement pattern itself.

Our approach is to help you focus on how your body moves instead of thinking about fixing your swing. The faults arise from bad movement patterns of the body caused by poor mobility.

Are you aware of how you stand, turn, and walk when you golf? All these movements have a huge impact on golf performance. Let's look at some of these swing errors and faults in a bit more detail.

The most common fault we see is the "slice." This is caused by the clubhead approaching from out-to-in across the intended target line with the clubface open to the swing path. The ball will start offline, traveling on a similar path as the clubhead—to the left for a right-handed golfer, to the right for a left-handed golfer, and then curve to the opposite direction. The open clubface imparts sidespin and hence curvature to the ball flight, resulting in the annoying slice. This shot is often caused by an incorrect swing sequence. The "slicer" starts the downswing sequence out of order, not leading with the lower body and hips, but rather by unwinding from the top of the swing, leading with the arms and shoulders. The club is swung out across the target line and then pulled back in toward the body on the downswing through the striking of the ball.

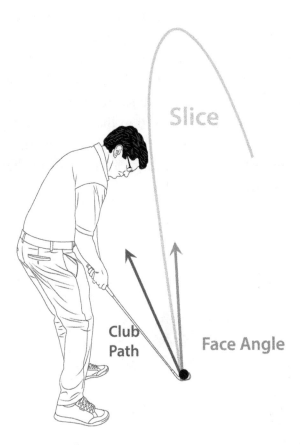

Improving the swing sequence will help eliminate this problem. Golfers who slice generally have very poor separation between the upper and lower body. Sometimes this is a learned technique and lack of coordination, but often they cannot turn well on the backswing with the upper body and then cannot lead with the lower body on the downswing. Typically, these golfers will have tight, immobile hips and limited upper-body mobility. They simply hack at the ball, chopping at it. They struggle with accuracy and also suffer from lack of distance.

The "hook" is another common fault and is the opposite shot shape of the slice. The clubhead path on the downswing approaches too much from inside the target line, and the clubface is closed to the swing path. So, for a right-handed golfer, the ball starts out to the right and then curves back to the left. For a left-handed golfer, it's the opposite.

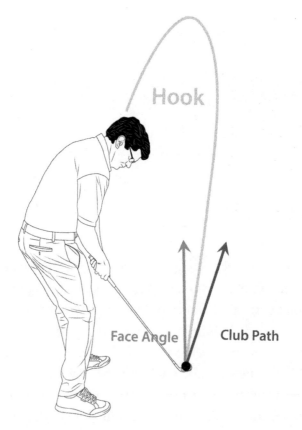

This is often caused by loss of posture. The golfer stands up or loses posture on the downswing. The hips move in toward the golf ball causing the clubhead path to come from the inside. Generally, this fault, as with the others, is caused by poor hip mobility and poor hip hinge mechanics. Golfers with tight hips cannot turn and pivot properly, and thus lose their posture during the swing.

Loss of clubhead speed is another very common swing fault. As we age, it is probably the number one problem for golfers. Sure, you're getting older, but that doesn't mean you need to lose speed—it can be maintained or even increased. What causes you to lose speed? The timing in the swing sequence is changing, the kinematic sequence is breaking down causing loss of speed.

Perhaps you're having trouble turning on the backswing, separating the upper body from the lower body and making that full backswing the way you used to. The backswing rotation is getting shorter. Declining posture may be causing restrictions in the thoracic spine and upper back. Unconsciously, over time, your shoulders slump forward, your posture slowly gets worse, and suddenly one season you can't turn. You can't make that full backswing anymore, and it's like "Hey, what the heck? I'm hitting it 10 yards shorter this year. What's going on? Must be my driver. Maybe I'm not swinging hard enough anymore." This was both of our stories ten years ago.

Your potential for speed is decreased because of the shorter backswing rotation, so you swing harder, trying to compensate for losing distance. But now you try to force the speed, hitting more with your arms and shoulders. This only makes it worse and you break the correct swing sequence (kinematic sequence). You start the downswing out of order. Instead of starting with the lower body, you are now trying to drive the power with your arms and shoulders. The upper body is leading on the downswing. The arms get ahead of the lower body pivot, and power cannot be transferred from the ground through the lower body to the clubhead. You end up "casting" the club, and that releases it too early. You not only lose speed, but the path of the swing will also be affected. So now swing direction, contact, and accuracy are more inconsistent.

To make this situation worse, you have the potential to get injured from swinging too hard to compensate for losing power. You could wrench and pull a muscle in your back or injure your wrist or shoulders from trying to power the club too much with the upper body. When you are not moving properly, you end up sore and tired after playing golf. It's not rugby or football, but sometimes it feels like it! Sound familiar? This is all caused, not by a technique issue, but by a lack of mobility, which then leads to the swing error. This compounds the problems and leads to injury. A progressively negative cycle is now started. This is no fun. But there is hope! The negative pattern can be interrupted and reversed by identifying the root cause— poor posture, which leads to declining body mobility.

Movement Patterns in Golf

There are several important movement patterns in golf, and the more you know about them, the better you'll understand the body-swing connection and how it can help your golf game.

Upper-Lower Body Separation

The interesting thing about golf is that your movement patterns in your swing are related to your swing thoughts. What does that mean? The scenarios below may help you understand. See if you can relate.

Susan is starting her backswing. Her hands and arms move first to start the backswing, but her torso and shoulders don't turn very well, neither do her hips. She isn't even aware of these limitations in her swing. Susan probably has some hip, shoulder and upper back restrictions preventing her from pivoting and making a good body turn on the backswing.

This will likely lead to her swaying and sliding her body back and forth to move the club. She can't turn very well because she has poor separation of the lower and upper body. Her hips and pelvis will slide from side to side. She might roll onto the outside of her back foot on the backswing with no body pivot and coil. She could even slide into a big, long backswing with her lead arm collapsing at the top of the backswing and the club wrapping around her head. On the downswing, she'll then slide her hips forward toward the target, rather than turning. She will throw her arms at the ball and probably be on her back foot at impact. She cannot extend her arms fully to strike the ball, her arms will bend up into her body, and she'll miss or top the ball.

Susan's golfing friends tell her, "Keep your head down!" She's got this thought burned into her brain. On the next swing … *thunk* … the club is hammered down into the ground behind the ball.

"Ouch, that hurts!" Susan exclaims. And the cycle repeats itself. Well, she kept her head down, that was her swing thought, but the real problem is that she can't rotate her body properly. Then her well-meaning friends tell her to keep her arms straight and shorten her backswing, but she simply can't change her technique. Frustrated, she blames herself.

"I'm a lousy golfer. This is no fun."

Sound familiar? Many golfers struggle with this. It's part of the body-swing connection.

Posture

Jim works in an office sitting behind a desk all day. He has been golfing for thirty years. When he sets up in his golf swing, his head is slumped forward and his back is rounded into the classic C-posture. This is a result of years of unconscious, poor posture. It's not great for golf (or daily living for that matter) and it's a hard position to swing the club from. Typically, golfers with this type of posture will suffer with more frequent neck pain and injuries. The deep neck flexors are weak from the slumping-head position. The chin is dropped down low and the head basically hinders the shoulders on the backswing. A good free shoulder turn is impossible. This posture position causes the upper chest muscles (pectorals) to be shortened, tight and weak. It also causes tight upper back muscles and weak lower back muscles. It limits the ability to turn and pivot properly on the backswing, which leads to loss of power, inconsistency, and back injury.

Over time, your body literally get glued into poor posture positions due to compressed connective tissue or "fascia". This is then carried over into the golf swing as well as other areas of your life. Golfers often look for quick fixes from chiropractors and massage therapists. Although these help to some degree, they are short-term fixes because we fall back into our negative habits and patterns. Until we look at ourselves and take responsibility for changing this, it will be much harder to improve our golf swing and feel better about ourselves.

Due to aging, fear, stress, and gravity our posture gets worse over time. You may not even be aware of your poor posture. But one morning, out of the blue, you wake up with a sore neck or back. Or you're at the top of your backswing and something tweaks, the pain goes shooting through your lower back. You wonder, *Where did that come from? I didn't do anything out of the ordinary, did I?* Well, you have been doing it to yourself for years, and your body decided that today was the day it had enough. You felt a tweak, you felt pain, your body is trying to tell you something. You need to listen to it!

Your posture is power. It has a positive effect on how much power your body can produce. If you look at all of today's great players in their golf posture, you will notice they look balanced and solid with great spine angles. If their daily posture wasn't good, they wouldn't be able to get their bodies into that address position.

When you have poor posture, your body has to compensate which then results in modifications in your movement. This can lead to diminished power as well as potential injury. Here are some common restrictions and limitations in your golf swing due to poor posture:

- Tight neck muscles cause reduced neck rotation making it difficult to maintain your spine angle.

- A weak core restricts your ability to transfer power from the lower body to the upper body. In addition, proper spine angle will not be maintained during the swing.

- Tight hamstrings make it difficult to achieve a good address position.

- Reduced range of motion in the hips leads to inconsistent swing patterns and lower back pain.

- Decreased torso rotation limits shoulder turn, causes poor sequencing between the lower and upper body and potentially causes back pain.

- Insufficient shoulder strength leads to decreased clubhead speed and poor club control.

In a nutshell, poor posture leads to headaches, shoulder issues, back pain, hip and knee issues, and foot problems. You get the picture ... it pretty much affects the entire body. The message here is to be mindful of your posture at all times as it will have a huge impact on your golf, your health, and your life.

Body Rotation

The easiest and most effective way to swing the club is based on the natural laws of motion and physics, using the rotational forces of gravity and centrifugal force to swing the golf club. In simple terms, it's the inertial force you feel pulling on the clubhead as you swing the club around your body. Being able to rotate and move the body in the correct sequence is the key to better golf.

It's not about using a special method or certain style of swing. It's about turning and pivoting your body effectively to harness and create centrifugal force to swing the golf club. This creates a flowing, consistent swing that generates effortless speed and accurate golf shots. When done right, it's like you're not even swinging the club. You get the club moving, you get your body moving and pivoting, and you simply get out of the way and let the club almost swing on its own. You set it in motion, and the inertia of the moving clubhead creates speed and keeps it on the correct path.

Throughout the swing, power and speed are transmitted from the ground up by way of the feet and the big muscles of the body—specifically the legs, pelvis, and back—

to the clubhead. At impact, your hands and arms transmit the speed and power, like cracking a whip. Hence, the correct rotation and sequence of rotation around a centered pivot is the key to easy, effortless speed and accuracy.

There is a definite correct sequence to the motion of swinging a golf club effectively. As we mentioned earlier, the measure of this motion—of the various moving parts of the body and the golf clubhead—is called the kinematic sequence. This is the fingerprint of your swing, or your signature of the movement of the club relative to your body. A trained instructor can look at a graph or printout of this signature and quickly determine if a player is a high-level player or an average golfer. Top-level players have a similar fingerprint or swing signature no matter how their swing looks. Let's review.

Generally, the correct sequence on the backswing is as follows:

1. clubhead moves first.
2. then the lead arm.
3. then the torso.
4. then the pelvis/hips.

On the downswing this sequence reverses:

4. pelvis/hips move first.
3. then the torso.
2. then the lead arm.
1. then the clubhead.

Refer to the kinematic sequence images at the beginning of this chapter.

This sequence creates maximum rotational force and transfer of that force and speed to the clubhead. It also creates consistency. Each moving segment of the swing, when moved in the correct order, will stabilize the swing and build speed and power, multiplying it to the next segment and finally applying it to the clubhead on the downswing through striking the golf ball. The key is to rotate around a fixed center, maintaining your spine tilt and posture, to help ensure accuracy and speed.

Good players easily rotate the upper body separately and independently from their lower body. This "separation of the rotation" creates effective, easy power.

The average golfer does not turn and pivot the body well due to limitations in their mobility, which often leads to swing faults and compensations to hit the golf ball. The result is inconsistent contact and poor golf. Improving your body rotation and swing sequence, and maintaining your posture will lead to better, more consistent golf.

Some key reference points are:

- In the setup position, generally, there is about 55-60 percent body weight and pressure on your front foot, with more weight on your heels and insteps of your feet, not the toes. You should be able to wiggle your toes in your shoes.

- As you turn on the backswing, about 75-80 percent of your body weight moves into your rear leg while some pressure is maintained on the front foot to help maintain a centered rotation.

- At top of the backswing, your upper body should be turned more than the hips, your back approximately 90 degrees to the target and your hips approximately turned 35 degrees, and the heel of the front foot may come slightly off the ground.

- Once the backswing is completed, the downswing is initiated from the ground up, the feet get active, front foot returns to its starting position, the feet press into the ground, the pelvis shifts, and hips begin to unwind.

- As the body unwinds on the downswing, there is a transfer of weight to the target foot. By the time the front arm is parallel to the ground on the downswing maximum pressure and force is now on the front foot and leg.

- From there, the hips continue unwinding, pulling the torso, shoulders, front arm, and finally the clubhead freewheeling through the ball.

- To complete the swing, you continue unwinding ending up facing the target with almost 100 percent of your body weight on the target foot, comfortably in balance.

Fixing the "Master" Faults

In this next section, we'll present some effective and simple drills that can help you overcome some of the common swing faults we discussed previously.

The "slice" is the most common swing fault, often caused by poor mobility and a poor swing sequence resulting in an out-to-in swing path on the downswing. The pattern with a slicer is that on the downswing the shoulders and upper body unwind out of sequence, moving first before the lower body and the club. The club path comes across the target path and body line with the clubface open and *boom*—a slice! Often the slicer is a very poor iron player as well. The ball may not slice as much with the irons because the club has more loft than woods, but it's basically the same swing pattern.

Golfers who slice need to work on mobility of the hips and upper body and retraining the body to move correctly. That's where proper golf instruction combined with mobility training works the best. The chronic slicer must work on the separation of the upper and lower body and retrain the two halves to work independently of each other, and in the correct sequence. This will help improve swing direction, ball flight, and consistency—and eliminate that slice permanently!

Inconsistent contact also plagues the average golfer. They hit the ball all over the clubface. They hit before the ball, commonly called hitting it "fat." The golf club bottoms out before the ball, a big divot is dug up, and the ball goes nowhere. Or they hit low on the blade, commonly called "topping" the ball or thin shots, and the ball flies as a low running grounder. These patterns can occur together and result from poor body rotation and loss of posture in the swing.

As we've said, good players have consistent posture and turn around a steady, fixed axis of rotation. From this, the common phrases "keep your head still" and "keep your eyes on the ball" came about. (Remember the scenario about Susan a few pages back?) This is a generalization meaning to keep a steady, centered axis of rotation. But most golfers don't really know or understand what "keeping your head still" and "eyes on the ball" means in terms of moving the body properly. Often they focus so much on a steady head position they don't turn their body.

To improve your game, think more about maintaining your posture during the swing around that centered axis. You need good mobility and flexibility to do this.

Try this. Stand up straight, feet hip-width apart, knees slightly bent. Now extend your arms out to the sides, parallel to the ground, palms down. With extended arms, rotate back and forth using your trunk and hips to turn, causing your arms to swing around you, keeping them level and your spine centered. Your head stays still because your spine, your center of axis, is staying centered and not swaying from side to side. This move is fairly easy for most people from a standing straight position.

Now tilt forward from the hips, mimicking your golf posture. Your arms are still extended in the helicopter position. Rotate your body so one hand points to the ground and the other is extended up behind you. Now try and rotate to the other side. This is much harder from the forward tilted spine position. You will feel stretching in your sides and lower back. Any restrictions you may have in your back and hips will now be apparent. Some of you may even feel some pain. Perhaps there may also be tightness in the back of the legs, the hamstrings and calves. Feel the difference once you are in the golf posture?

What happens to many golfers from this forward tilted starting position, due to mobility and technique issues, is they stand up in the backswing, rising out of their starting position as they take the club back. Then on the downswing, they might lunge at the ball rather than turning. Or they will stand up as they go into the ball on the forward swing, pulling up and away from the ball. Or they will do both. The result is the center of the swing is moving up and down too much relative to the original starting position of the body and golf ball. The club will bottom out in different spots relative to the ball. The unskilled eye will see the head moving up and down, hence the phrase "keep your head down," but not realize the head is the symptom and not the cause.

Another common swing fault related to poor posture (but not talked about much because it's harder to see) is called "early extension." It's the silent killer of golf swings! Basically, with early extension, your pelvis rises and moves closer to the ball on the downswing; you lose your posture as the lower body stands up rather than rotating on the down swing. A good way to picture this is imagine you were sitting on a chair toward the edge of the seat; you're at the top of your backswing. As you swing forward on the downswing you would rise up off the chair.

Early extension is caused primarily by poor hip mobility; this results in limited rotation of the pelvis on the downswing. The problem with early extension is you are getting closer to the ball with your pelvis as you lose posture on the downswing, but the ball is not moving, so compensations must occur to make contact with the ball. A whole host of swing issues then occur. About 70 percent of amateurs lose their posture and early extend in the swing. With Tour players it's less than 1 percent. Maintaining your posture in the golf swing is critical for playing good golf.

You can try to "fix" your technique, do some swing drills, and take lessons, which may help in the short term, but if you don't deal with the underlying mobility issues and body rotation patterns, your success of getting a fix will be elusive. Working on your swing sequence and mobility will eliminate many faults without even dealing with the technique issues.

There are some simple golf movement tests you can do to help determine your level of mobility restrictions and make you more aware of the body-swing connection. Below are a few tests we use from the Titleist Performance Institute (TPI), the world's leading educational organization devoted to the study of how the human body moves and functions in relation to the golf swing. Their research is based on studying thousands of golfers, from Tour players to average golfers. We are both TPI certified for functional movement assessment of golfers.

Toe Touch

Being able to touch your toes is a good indicator of overall body mobility and physical health. For your golf game, touching your toes means you'll be able to hinge your hips, which is important for proper setup in the golf swing. Some people simply can't touch their toes due to injuries or back problems, but for most it's the result of restrictions in the hips, lower back, and backs of the legs.

According to TPI, about 40 percent of all amateur golfers have difficulty touching their toes, while over 80 percent of Tour players can touch their toes.

The toe touch test is simple to perform. Stand with feet together, toes facing directly forward. Bend from the hips and touch the ends of your fingers to the tips of your toes without bending your knees. Perform the test without warming up.

Seated Trunk Rotation

This is a good test to identify how much rotational mobility you have in the thoracic spine (upper back area) and determines how well and easily you can turn the upper body. Many golfers lack true thoracic mobility and as a result have difficulty turning on the backswing properly. Ribcage restrictions and poor upper body posture contribute greatly to this.

Sit tall on a bench or end of a chair with feet together flat on the floor. Place a club or dowel in your hands with arms extended out in a "W" position, shoulders pulled back and relaxed. Now try to turn back and forth, testing your end range of motion in each direction while keeping the feet flat and knees together.

Golfers with restrictions find this test difficult and will cheat and lean to each side rather than turn. Minimum rotation in each direction should be 45 degrees.

About 90 percent of Tour players can turn greater than 50 degrees in each direction, while only 60 percent of amateurs can turn this far. Tour players simply turn and pivot better!

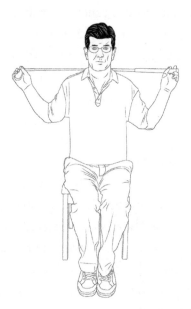

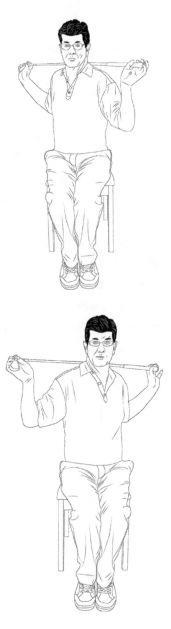

Pelvic/Torso Rotation

These tests measure your ability to separate your body rotation and turn your upper body and pelvis independently of each other, which is critical for turning effectively in the golf swing.

Set up in your golf posture, tilted forward, with arms crossed over your chest, hands on your shoulders. First, try to rotate your pelvis back and forth without moving the upper body or sliding your hips. Now try to rotate the upper body torso without moving the pelvis and lower body.

You should have smooth easy rotations back and forth in each body area when performing each test separately, with no shaking, grimacing, pain, swaying, or sliding.

The range of motion is not what is measured, but rather whether you can separate the rotation of the pelvis/lower body from the thoracic/upper body.

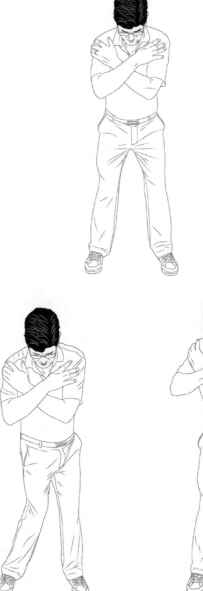

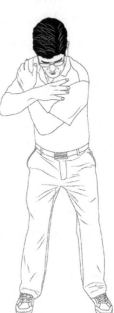

Difficulty in performing the above tests indicates thoracic and lumbar spine restrictions with hip mobility issues. Both are key areas for swinging the golf club effectively.

There are many different types of drills and exercises golfers can do to fix specific swing faults but they are too numerous to mention all of them here; that's another book on its own!

What we find is that many golfers simply don't spend enough time improving their overall mobility and posture. And they don't spend enough time working on their golf swing body rotation, and swing sequence. Instead, they are looking for those "quick swing fixes."

Movement Drills

We've stated repeatedly that rotating effectively and efficiently is one of the master keys to better golf. A good place to start is with simple and effective mobility drills for golf, several examples are provided below. We've found them to be some of the best and simplest drills to help your overall mobility and improve your golf swing technique at the same time. These drills are dynamic, designed to get you moving, and easy and fun to do. They don't require you to hit golf balls, so you can do them anywhere you have room to move and swing a club. They can be incorporated easily into your warmup and practice routines.

Standing Helicopter Turns

Stand erect with feet hip-width apart, feet pointing straight forward. Stretch arms out from sides parallel to the ground, palms down, fingertips stretched out. Turn and rotate trunk from side to side to move the arms, feet stay flat on the ground, hips may turn but not sway. The feeling is the trunk rotating to move the arms, not the arms swinging to rotate the trunk. Do ten to fifteen reps each side.

Thoracic Golf Swing Turns

Stand erect, hold your driver upside down in front of you as a support stick with your left hand on top of driver head to balance you. Hold the driver far enough away from your body so your left arm is stretched out straight and you are bent over slightly, similar to your golf posture. Let your right arm hang down in front of you. Then rotate and turn your torso to the right side and swing the right hand and arm up over your right shoulder as high as you can. Keep the left hand on top of the driver for support while you look forward. The feeling you want is a rotation of the upper spine, the chest and ribcage, not a sliding in the hips. Do five to ten reps each side.

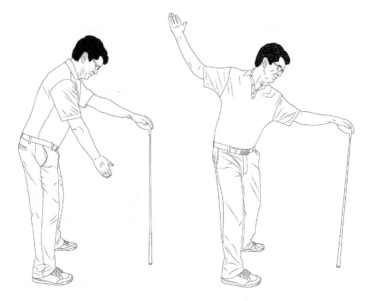

"Hello There, Target" Finish Drill

Stand erect with feet hip width apart, hold a club out in front of you with your trail hand (right if right-handed golfer, left if left-handed golfer), arm comfortably extended, grip end of club pressing lightly against the middle of your body, bodyweight approximately 50/50 between both legs. Now rotate to face an imaginary target. The club moves because you turn to face the target. The gip end stays touching your body; arm position and club position have not changed from your starting position. You finish in full natural height, hips and trunk facing the target. 100 percent of your body weight is on your target foot to finish the motion. This exercise teaches you to move your weight and the club with your body rotation toward the target.

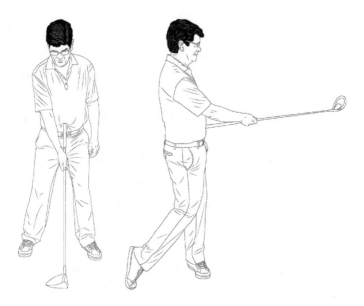

Golf Pivot Hands on Hips

This is like the "Hello There, Target" Finish Drill, except you are not holding a club. Stand in your starting golf stance, hands on hips, knees slightly bent, weight balanced toward the heels of the feet with more pressure on your lead side than the trail side leg. Your lead foot is flared out slightly toward the target, the trail foot is square to the target line. Rotate your hips about 30 degrees toward the trail leg, enough to move your weight onto that leg. From this position, rotate your hips toward the target, finishing with your hips and trunk squarely facing your target. All your weight should finish on your lead leg with your trail foot rotated up on the toes, perpendicular to the ground. Your knees stay slightly flexed during the motion, and the lead leg knee straightens naturally as you turn to finish.

The rotation of the hips and body is what moves and transfers your body weight. This exercise may be difficult for those who don't rotate very well and swing primarily with their arms.

Repeat this move on the other side. Don't worry if you feel awkward and unbalanced. This will help your hip mobility in both directions and improve your balance and athleticism. Practice this exercise regularly, ten to twenty reps at a time, and with your eyes closed! Use it as a warm-up and training drill.

Golf Pivot with Club Behind Shoulders in Golf Posture
Stand in your golf stance, knees slightly bent, driver behind your neck on your shoulders, arms extended in 'W' position, with shoulders pulled back slightly. Turn your torso to the top of the backswing position until your upper torso rotates to at least 90 degrees (or as far as your mobility allows). The grip end of the golf club will point toward the ground as you maintain your starting posture position with your head centered, looking directly at the ground. You should feel a stretch in your upper back muscles as you turn. From this top of backswing position, unwind with your hips to your finish position. Practice good rotation form. The feeling of this movement is a balanced centered rotation of the body. On the backswing, the upper body pivots more than the hips. The forward motion is an unwinding from the ground up led by the hips. This is a good swing practice drill and warm up

exercise. Incorporate it regularly into your golf practice routine.

Split Grip Thoracic Rotation Drill

In your golf stance, hold a driver like a hockey stick with your hands apart, lead hand at the top of the grip, trail hand below the grip in the middle of the shaft. Do some practice golf swings. Focus on a full body rotation on the backswing with a good thoracic turn, letting your lead heel come off the ground. Pump the club to the top of the backswing position a few times, then do your transition move making sure the lead heel and foot return to their starting positions for the downswing. The forward motion begins from the ground up. You should feel pressure and weight on the lead foot early into the downswing motion. The forward rotation and turn are with your weight moving from your trail leg to the lead foot and leg. Unwind to a full complete finish. Try to not let the club shaft touch your body on the forward swing. This is a good drill for overall golf swing body rotation. It allows you to feel the correct sequence of motion on the downswing.

Swish Drill

Stand in your golf posture. Hold the golf club with your hands near the clubhead instead of the grip end. The focus is on swinging the club and making it *swish* in the air as loud as you can, like cracking a whip. This is a good drill for promoting wrist mobility, as your wrists will unhinge freely back and forth. It takes tension out of the hands while holding the club, giving you softer hand pressure, and it also helps you feel the correct sequence of motion for the downswing. To make it *swish*, your lower body instinctively leads on the downswing, and the club is released to catch up. You want to hear the sound as late as possible in the downswing.

Stepping Drill for Swing Sequence

This is a good drill for promoting correct sequence of motion in the golf swing. You can use any club, but a middle iron like a 6 or 7 works best. Take your starting golf stance and use tees or other objects to mark your foot positions. As you start your backswing, step back with your lead foot toward your trail foot. Then return your lead foot to the marked starting position as you start the downswing and rotate to finish from there. (Kind of like stepping into hitting with a baseball bat.) Remember the correct sequence of motion: club first on the backswing, lower body first on the downswing. Start slow. It might be harder than you think, especially for those who move out of sequence in their swing! Begin this drill without hitting balls then progress to hitting balls.

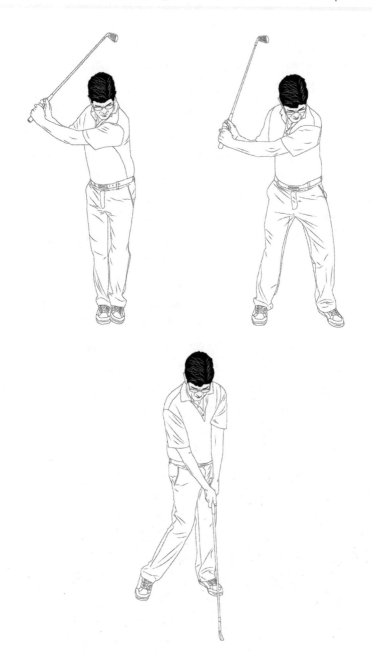

Half Swing Drill with Golf Club

Set up in your golf stance with a 6 or 7 iron. Place two tees in the ground about the width of the clubhead. Give yourself a little extra room to swing the clubhead through the tees back and forth. Move the club halfway back, feeling the correct sequence of motion for the backswing along with the movement of your body weight from lead foot to trail foot. The club at halfway back is parallel to your intended target line, toe of the clubhead up, lead arm comfortably extended, trail arm folding, hands passive, no change in wrist angles or grip formation.

The forward swing is then initiated by the lower body; your weight moves to lead foot on the forward swing as you let the club swing between the two tees and you finish with all your body weight on your lead foot and leg, with hips and torso facing the target. The club is now extended in front of you, a mirror image of halfway back position. The trail arm is comfortably extended, lead arm folded, hands are passive, no change in wrist angles or grip formation, toe of the clubhead is up.

Swinging the club between the tees gives you feedback for the direction of the clubhead. Keep your focus on the body rotation, moving the club back and forth. You will find with practice that you are not directing the club between the tees; it simply happens as a result of the swing motion. Half swings are a fantastic way to work on full swing motion.

This drill can be done anywhere you have room to swing halfway back and through, indoors or outdoors.

You do not need golf balls. Progress to hitting golf balls once you can easily let the clubhead swing consistently between the tees.

Barry's Story

As we get older, we tend to naturally expect some level of mobility restrictions, but these can really occur at any age, and golf will be a struggle. I've seen it in some of my students in their twenties and thirties that are seemingly fit and strong but have underlying body restrictions and limitations. One of my students, Jason, is in his early thirties. Before he came to me, he had been playing for a few years, bouncing around taking lessons, watching YouTube video after YouTube video, and not getting anywhere. Jason was really struggling with his golf game and not able to break 100. He was totally frustrated and couldn't understand why he wasn't getting better. Once we started working together, I was able to assess him and discover the mobility problems that were affecting his golf motion and inability to maintain his golf posture. I moved him out of thinking the golf swing was a about a series of isolated positions and more into thinking about it as movement patterns. The lightbulb went on! He began to really understand how the swing positions were a result of the body motion and correct swing sequence, and to have a correct swing sequence he needed to work on his mobility. Everything changed for him. He improved fast and dramatically, taking 20 strokes off his golf game in one season! You are never too young or too old to see positive and amazing results when you focus on movement patterns and freeing up your body.

Chapter 5:

Mind-Body Connection

Controlling the breath is a prerequisite to controlling the mind and the body.

–Swami Rama, *Science of Breath: A Practical Guide*

Some of you may have heard the phrase "mind-body connection" before, but what is the mind-body connection and how will it help your golf game? Well, it's quite simple. The mind-body connection means that what we think, feel, and believe can have a positive or negative effect on how our body functions physiologically. It can affect the health of our bodies and how we perform.

At the same time, the foods we eat, how much we exercise, and even our posture and breathing can affect our mental state both positively and negatively. This produces a complex and interconnected relationship between our mind and body.

We're going to look at a few areas of the mind-body connection and how they impact your golf. Specifically, we'll look at breathing, posture, fascia (connective tissue), visualization, and meditation.

Breathe for Better Golf

Believe it or not, proper breathing is one of the best ways to improve your golf game. Breathing is the essence of life. You can live for weeks without food and three to five days without water, but you can only live for a few minutes without oxygen. Becoming as efficient as possible at breathing can make golf and life better. Those who can control their breath in a certain way can better control their mind and body. And it helps you create a habit of positive thinking.

Do you pay attention to how you are breathing on the golf course? When you are under stress or in fear of missing that three-foot putt, do you sometimes hold your breath and are not even aware of it? During your swing, do you hold your breath, bracing yourself for that shot of pain in your back or hips on the follow-through? Do your upper chest muscles tighten?

The power and benefits of proper breathing, particularly diaphragmatic breathing, have been experienced by yogis, Buddhists, and swamis for thousands of years. Modern medical science is just catching up and beginning to understand that breath is the essential link between general wellness and the mind-body connection. Swami Rami, one of the great Himalayan Yogi Masters and founder of the Himalayan Institute made this concept mainstream in his classic guide, *Science of Breath*. His remarkable feats of controlling his breath, body temperature, stopping and controlling his heart, psychic abilities, and mind control were much studied in scientific laboratories in the late '60s and early '70s. More recently, Wim Hof, a Dutch extreme athlete, also known as the Iceman, has shown similar feats using his unique method of breathing, which result in a multitude of benefits for human health.

You breathe over twenty-three thousand times a day. That's a lot of breathing! And you do this automatically. Breathing is the only vital body function that is both involuntary (done without conscious thought) and voluntary (within your thought control). Understanding and practicing proper conscious breathing will help you control your autonomic nervous system (which looks after involuntary functions, those you don't have to think about). This can give you a huge competitive advantage over others in golf, in terms of stamina and focus.

There are various theories to explain what happens under pressure to athletes and those in high-stress situations. Some rise to the occasion and achieve greatness while others collapse or "choke," blowing leads and likely victories, freezing up as if in a life or death situation. In these circumstances, the fight-or-flight response kicks in. It is hard-wired into your brain and body and expressed through your fascia (connective tissue) in your body.

Your breathing gets shallow, the brain releases cortisol or adrenaline under pressure, there is sudden loss of coordination and fine motor function, thinking becomes foggy, and even vision gets worse. Suddenly it all changes and becomes an altered state of non-performance. Does this sound familiar?

Thankfully, there's something that can help control the mind and body during stress, and that is diaphragmatic breathing. Focusing on breathing with your diaphragm keeps your mind in the present moment. It gives you a task to focus on, distracting you from the fear and anxiety of the "what if" future. You have a chance to maintain being in the moment while under pressure to perform.

Your diaphragm is a large plate of muscle across the midsection of your body, attached to your lower ribs. Your heart and lungs are located above the diaphragm muscle and your abdominal organs are situated below it. As you breathe in, the lungs inflate, filling with air, and the diaphragm muscle moves downward, causing the belly to expand. As you breathe out, the diaphragm comes back up, and the belly falls back to normal.

Diaphragmatic breathing activates the parasympathetic nervous system (part of the autonomic nervous system), which calms you and allows you to slow down, to control your rhythm and tempo, and maintain your fine motor skills. It helps keep your thinking clear, preventing "brain fog" caused by lack of oxygen. We've all had those disappointing rounds where after we unwind and debrief, we say, "What was I thinking?" Diaphragmatic breathing will help you to make better decisions when under stress in your game, it's the mind-body connection in action.

The brain uses about 20 percent of the oxygen taken in even though it comprises only about 2 percent of body weight. About 70 percent of a body's toxins are released through breath. Unfortunately, many people do not breathe properly, they take sips of air and hold their breath during times of tension and anxiety. It's been estimated that over 90 percent of the population uses just 30 percent of their actual lung capacity. We are shortchanging our lives through poor breathing habits!

It's difficult to perform at your best, both on and off the golf course, if you are not breathing properly. Breathing efficiently fully fills your lungs with oxygen which is then transported to your cells to feed and clean them. Your cells are organized into muscle, bone, tissue, and organs, and allow you to perform every necessary bodily function. If you don't get the proper amount of oxygen into your lungs, you can't feed your cells. If you can't feed your cells, your body can't function properly. So you can see how proper breathing is vital for your health and your performance on the golf course, and it's totally within your control!

Diaphragmatic breathing requires you to be conscious of your breathing. It enables your lungs to absorb much more oxygen. Your cells constantly need a new supply of oxygen to produce higher levels of energy, which allows you to think, create, and perform at an optimal level. The combination of increased oxygen combined with proper posture form the foundation for you to play better golf and have better health.

Picture a newborn baby lying in a crib. Their belly moves up and down gently as they breathe. They breathe that way instinctively. This is diaphragmatic breathing. But what happens over time, due to fear, aging, stress, and anxiety, is that many people start to breathe using the muscles of their upper chest. These muscles get tight, sore, and exhausted. They take in shallow breaths. Not enough oxygen gets into their cells, which can lead to many health problems. To be the most effective at feeding your cells, you need to breathe using your diaphragm.

Practice diaphragmatic breathing for five to ten minutes every day to make it a habit. This will have huge benefits to you as a golfer. It helps to get more blood and oxygen into your cells, giving you more energy to move better. It releases toxins and negative emotions from your cells. It has a calming effect, allowing you to stay relaxed under pressure, especially on the tee before you take that first swing. It will help steady your nerves when making that 3-foot putt to save par. It opens your rib cage, and as a result you turn better. Your diaphragm muscle gets stronger, which strengthens your core. This helps with your golf rotation. You'll have more sustained energy, so you won't have that fifteenth hole slump and start making mistakes. Better breathing leads to better focus and concentration, which is absolutely necessary for playing good golf. And the most amazing thing is that all these benefits can be transferred to everyday life!

Before we started the practice of diaphragmatic breathing, we were both often winded and out of energy by the thirteenth or fourteenth hole. We needed a late-round energy boost to get us through to the eighteenth hole. What made this situation worse was we were relatively young and neither of us smoked. But we both worked at jobs that were very stressful. When we look back, we realize now that we were not breathing properly. We were taking in shallow breaths, using the muscles of our upper chests. Sometimes we would be holding our breath without even realizing it. Once we discovered diaphragmatic breathing, everything changed for us. Getting to the eighteenth hole with energy to spare was a breeze. It calmed us under pressure and made our golf game more enjoyable overall. We felt so much better. When you feel better, you have more fun.

In *USA Today*, November 2018, PGA Tour player Bryson DeChambeau discussed how diaphragmatic breathing aided his training and digestion, and the week following that article he won the Las Vegas Shriners PGA Tour event for his fifth career win since joining the tour in 2017. Since then, he's won two more times, including the 2020 U.S. Open. How's that for the positive impact of diaphragmatic breathing on golf performance!

There have been many studies that have documented the benefits of diaphragmatic breathing; they are summarized below:

- It increases your energy by improving oxygen levels in your bloodstream, the essential nutrient for your body's cells.

- It improves the respiratory system, strengthens the diaphragm and core, opens the rib cage, and releases tension in the chest, allowing for better posture and breathing. It helps stabilize your core.
- It activates the parasympathetic nervous system (the rest and digest part of the nervous system). This is the opposite of the fight-or-flight response of the sympathetic nervous system.
- It helps relieve stress and anxiety. Poor breathing is present in 83 percent of people suffering from anxiety. They breathe shallowly, using the muscles of the upper chest.
- It improves and strengthens the lymphatic system, which depends on gravity and muscle movement for body cleansing. Diaphragmatic breathing can be an important part of keeping everything moving, protecting the body from viruses, bacteria, infection, and other threats.
- It releases muscle tension. When we experience anger, frustration, or pain, our breathing becomes shallow, our bodies tense. Diaphragmatic breathing helps counter this.
- It improves the cardiovascular system. It increases circulation to the heart, liver, and brain by massaging those organs. There is a strong correlation between poor breathing habits and heart attacks. One study found 100 percent of heart attack victims did not know about

or practice diaphragmatic breathing. Another study found that those in recovery who practiced diaphragmatic breathing with various forms of exercise and meditation had 50 percent less incidence of another heart attack after five years.

- It enhances the digestive system and can improve irritable bowel syndrome, constipation, and stomach disorders (all of which are related to stress and anxiety).

- It improves skin tone, slows premature aging, and reduces wrinkles by reducing stress and moving toxins from the fascia at the cellular level. There's a reason why smokers look older—a lack of sufficient oxygen!

- It gives the brain plenty of oxygen for optimal performance and a general feeling of wellness. Improved oxygen flow to the brain helps achieve clarity, creates a feeling of well-being, facilitates productivity, and generally improves negative thinking. It's one thing to think positive, but you also have to breathe positive! There's that mind-body connection again.

Our key message here is that proper diaphragmatic breathing is vital for improving your golf performance, particularly if you are dealing with the stress of competitive golf. But it's also necessary for a healthy life. Stress and anxiety are killers and performance inhibitors. Common stressors in life—worrying about work, family, health, and finances—if not managed properly, will shorten your life and make you miserable! Never mind trying to improve your golf and enjoy yourself on the course. Learning to breathe properly is fundamental to living well.

Diaphragmatic Breathing Technique

Below is a simple way for you to begin the habit of diaphragmatic breathing. Practice this technique for at least ten minutes every day and notice how it makes you feel.

- Lie in a comfortable position and place your hands on your belly.

- Inhale through your nose slowly and deeply into your abdomen, feeling your belly rise under your hand. Your upper chest should not move much. At the end of the inhale, take a slight pause.

- Then slowly exhale through the nose, feeling your belly sink under your hands. Squeeze every last bit of air out, feeling as if your navel is getting drawn down to your spine.

- Continue with these slow deep breaths, inhaling and exhaling. Feel the movement of your belly rising and falling as air flows in and out of your lungs. Enjoy the slow rhythm of your breath as it relaxes you.

- Practice this breathing for at least ten minutes at a time. When you're ready, give your body a nice stretch and get up. You will feel great!

Try this diaphragmatic breathing technique next time you're feeling that afternoon lag. Instead of reaching for a coffee, a sugary drink, or snack, do some deep diaphragmatic breathing for a few minutes. If you can't lie down, you can do this technique sitting. Sit tall with good posture and engage in some deep breathing, filling the lungs deeply, inhaling and exhaling through the nose. Fill your body with oxygen and re-energize.

Power up with Posture

As you know by now, good posture is critically important for your golf game. But being conscious of your posture should have started long before you came anywhere near a golf club or took up the game of golf. Poor posture does not occur overnight, it's the result of years of being unconscious to how you stand, sit, and move. The biggest physical challenge faced by amateur golfers entering their fifties is the poor posture they've developed over the past twenty to thirty years.

What we see in many middle-aged people is that they do not stand properly. They slouch forward with their feet splayed out like a duck, their rib cage is collapsed into their core and their head is slumped forward. They also shift their weight to one side, hyperextending their knee on that side. This causes a lot of compression and misalignment in the body. There are many negative effects on the body because of poor posture:

- Overly tight, shortened hip muscles, which tug your upper body forward and disrupt your posture.
- Tightened chest muscles, which pull your shoulders forward.
- Weak core muscles, which tips your body forward and can put you off balance.
- Cellulite, arthritis in the joints, plantar fasciitis, and restless leg syndrome.
- Headaches, shoulder issues, back pain, and joint pain.

When the upper chest collapses inward to the core, the belly displaces outward. Many people develop a belly or a "spare tire" as they age. They think it's too much fat around the middle and work hard to get rid of it. But if they continue with poor posture, that will make it impossible. And it's not necessarily too much fat, but rather displaced fascia (connective tissue) from the collapse of the ribcage into the core.

The primary reason for this is many people are not conscious of their posture. They don't think about it on a daily basis. They don't remind themselves to sit, stand and walk tall.

Let's look at good posture. The following describes how to put your body into proper postural alignment:

- Stand tall with feet slightly apart, directly under the hip joints, toes facing forward.
- Chin is slightly tucked so it is parallel to the floor.

- Shoulders are even (roll your shoulders up, back, and down to help achieve this).
- Neutral spine (no flexing or arching to over-emphasize the curve in your lower back).
- Arms are at your sides with elbows straight and even.
- Abdominal muscles are braced.
- Hips are even.
- Knees are even and pointing straight ahead, but not hyperextended (locked).
- Body weight is distributed evenly on both feet.
- About 60 percent of your body weight is on your heels.

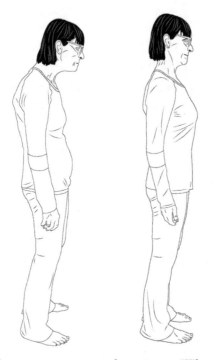

Check your posture in the mirror. What do you see? Quick posture checks can help you become more aware of asymmetries in your body and areas you need to address. Begin to pay more attention to your posture and make it a habit to check your postural alignment daily.

A good way to develop proper postural habits is by using a technique called "rooting" which we learned from Deanna Hansen, the founder of Block Therapy. It puts your body into proper alignment and helps increase your core strength. It's similar to the good posture description above but with a few tweaks. Once you get into this position, you'll feel immediate relief just standing there. The aim is to practice rooting every day for five to ten minutes until it becomes a habit. Here's how to perform rooting:

- Stand with your feet together, facing forward, equal weight on both feet, feet directly below the hip joints.
- Knees are soft (slightly bent). Avoid locked or hyperextended knees, as this causes the pelvis to tilt and the belly to fall.
- Place a thick book wrapped in a towel (approximately 3 inches thick) up high between your inner thighs and squeeze the book. (We use a wooden tool called a "block buddy" that you'll hear more about later.) When our bodies become accustomed to improper posture, we lose the integration of the inner thigh (adductor) muscles. Strong adductors are very important for a proper foundation.
- Arms are at your sides, palms facing forward.
- Chin slightly tucked so the head is properly balanced on the neck.
- Squeeze your butt cheeks (this slightly shifts the pelvis forward).
- Stand this way for two to three minutes while breathing from your diaphragm.
- Envision yourself growing roots into the ground and feeling more stable.

This technique helps to align the pelvis and create the proper foundation when standing or sitting. It creates stability and strength and helps prevent falling or torqueing out of alignment.

The rooting technique, if practiced for five or ten minutes every day, will have a profound impact on your health and golf performance because of the proper postural alignment it brings to your body. Even if you don't have a block buddy or book handy, you can still practice this anytime throughout the day by just getting into position and squeezing your butt cheeks, and holding the squeeze while you breathe from your diaphragm.

Tammy's Story

I have always thought of myself as a reasonably healthy and fit person. I played decent golf throughout my thirties into my fifties. But I worked at a desk job, and it took its toll on me, although I didn't realize it at the time. I remember waking up one morning in my mid-forties, and I couldn't turn my neck. I was in excruciating pain! What the heck happened? I took some Tylenol to help ease the pain, but there was no relief.

I was attending the Canadian Women's National Golf Championship the following week and was quite concerned about how I would play. As anticipated, the pain was terrible, so I took more pain killers and pushed through it. I played dreadful. There happened to be a massage therapist at the event for the players, so I went to see her. During the massage, she said, "Your neck and shoulders are a mess! You need major work done. You shouldn't even be golfing this week."

I realized then that I had not been conscious of my posture for a long time. The stress and pressure of my job had taken away my focus on my health. My body was trying to tell me something! When I got back home, I immediately found an excellent massage therapist. She was good! Even so, it took almost nine months (and a lot of money) to get my neck and shoulders somewhat back to normal. The culprit that led to all this pain and suffering was years of poor posture sitting at a desk. I'm now so much more conscious of my posture, and with my self-care fascia release technique (you'll hear about this in the next section), my neck pain has never come back.

You can see that proper posture is essential for golf. You must be able to put your body into the proper posture at address and maintain it throughout the golf swing so you can make good contact with the ball. You should also have proper posture for everyday health. The benefits are numerous:

- Reduced lower back pain.
- Fewer headaches.
- Increased energy levels.
- Less tension in your shoulders and neck.
- Reduced muscle fatigue.
- Decreased risk of joint damage.
- Improved circulation and digestion.
- Increased confidence.

Practice good posture every day, become more conscious of how you sit, stand and walk. It will have a very positive effect on the mind-body connection. It will help your golf, your health, and your life.

Find Fascia Fitness

So far we've shared our techniques for breathing and posture that will noticeably improve your golf game. But the secret sauce that pulls this all together is releasing compressed fascia in your body. Fascia is the fibrous connective tissue in your body that encloses, separates, and penetrates every muscle, nerve, artery, vein, and organ in your body. It's the structure that holds everything together. It stores and moves water and carries energy. It also carries your emotions and has many nerve endings. Some say it's the vehicle through which your essence, your source energy, your spirit, or whatever you may call it, travels.

Fascia has a direct connection to pain in your body. Chronic pain is the accumulation of many factors over a lifetime. It is what you do all the time, every day, that really determines how your body functions and moves. How you sit, stand, walk, and even sleep impacts your health. Aging, gravity, poor posture, disease, surgery, and illness create compression and adhesions in the fascia deep inside your body. This results in pain and tension. Blood and oxygen cannot flow through the adhesions freely, so the cells within the compressed tissues cannot function properly. This causes restrictions in your mobility; you lose flexibility, you have joint issues, poor circulation, and pain from compression on the nerves. Fascia can seal with a force of up to 2000 pounds per square inch so that pain is very difficult to release!

Pain caused by compressed fascia can be tough to address because the cause site for the pain is not always where the pain is felt. To understand what causes pain and find the compressed tissue deep inside the body to release it can be a challenge. For example, take back pain—it's likely the hips, legs, abdomen, and rib cage that must be addressed to release tension in the back. The compression that occurs over time in the front of the body can cause the vertebrae to misalign; the discs compress and bulge, putting pressure on the nerve roots, causing pain, and creating intense muscle fatigue.

We have discovered a unique self-care bodywork practice called Block Therapy that releases compressed fascia deep within the body. The amazing thing about this technique is that it's a therapy, exercise, and meditation all in one modality. We us a therapeutic wooden tool called a "block buddy" to sink deeply into the tissue, bringing increased blood flow and oxygen into the area, warming the adhesions and melting the powerful seal between the layers of restricted fascia. Combined with the diaphragmatic breathing and postural awareness training we discussed earlier, this practice brings a whole new level of awareness and health to your body at the cellular level.

Lower back pain is a very common problem for many golfers and is cited as the second most frequent reason to visit a doctor. The socioeconomic impact of chronic lower back pain is massive. The American Physical Therapy Association website says that "More than one-third of adults say low back pain has affected their ability to engage in tasks of daily living, exercise, and sleep. More than half (54 percent) of Americans who experience low back pain spend the majority of their workday sitting. When experiencing low back pain, nearly three in four of Americans use pain medication as a way to relieve their symptoms."

Barry's Story

I remember the first time I saw it.

"A block of wood! Are you kidding me? That's going to fix my back?" A lifetime of struggling with back pain, mobility issues, negative emotions, and fear was melted away by that piece of wood! I remember so vividly when I was introduced to the "block" about seven years ago. Tammy and I were at her brother's house for Christmas Eve, and his girlfriend had this piece of wood and was getting into this strange new fascia release therapy.

She said, "Just lie on it, it will help your back." I was struggling mightily at the time with back pain and was desperate enough to try it. Of course, I did it all wrong. I laid my back directly on it thinking that was how to use it, because all my other therapies focused on the back. It almost killed me! I could barely get up from lying on that piece of wood the first time, but I was intrigued. So was Tammy, as she had some lingering sports-related injuries.

We were intrigued enough to follow-up with the founder of this technique, Deanna Hansen, to learn more. I was skeptical but desperate, and so I booked a session with her. After that first therapy session, relief was fast, not overnight, but it made sense and positive changes were quick. This was the first therapy that actually dealt with the root cause, not just the pain site. That's what makes it unique. I had one of those "aha" moments for my back pain and have not looked back since.

As you know, I'm a PGA of Canada golf professional, and have suffered most of my adult life with daily back pain and mobility issues. This is from a lifetime of traumas, sports injuries, and general repetitive golf motion strain, all of which culminated in the classic golfer lumbar L5-S1 disk herniation. No one could seem to solve or explain my general pain and mobility issues. I was told I was just stiff, that it's genetics, injury, just plain ol' getting old, and general mechanical dysfunction, whatever that is. Things got a lot worse after the disk herniation. I had constant sciatic pain; sitting, standing, walking, resting, sleeping, and general life was painful, never mind trying to play golf! The daily back stiffness, lower back compression, and pain were wearing me out. I was aging fast, putting on weight, and also carrying around the extra baggage of negative emotions and fear.

The negativity of prolonged pain and injury is like living with a slow poison in your system, slowly draining you of life. All the physical therapies and training I did, from chiropractic to physiotherapy, yoga, sports training, and exercise, provided temporary relief. But nothing lasted until I found that block of wood.

Fast forward a few years—my daily pain is gone, and I'm not on medication of any kind, not even over-the-counter stuff. And I'm off my big crux—self-medicating with too much alcohol. I'm so grateful for my new lease on life. I've gone from a ballooning 40-inch waist to now pushing a 34-inch waist, like back when I was thirty! I feel and look twenty years younger, and I'm 25 pounds lighter. I've also shed all that negative baggage and fear I carried around for years through the help of this new fascia release therapy.

That block of wood is now part of my daily living. It complements everything I do. It's not a huge time commitment either. It only takes a few minutes every day to change your life forever. Because of block therapy, I'm more health conscious and able to live a fit, positive life, and still play great golf!

Albert Einstein said coincidences are God's way of staying anonymous. I'm so grateful I gave that piece of wood a try on that fateful day. Tammy is now trained and certified is this technique, and we teach it to others. Amazing to think a block of wood could be so life-changing!

See What You Want ... and Get It

Imagination is everything, it's the preview of life's coming attractions.

–Albert Einstein

Often, we imagine the worst situations before they ever happen. We visualize our fears rather than best-case scenarios. For example, you're playing in an event. You have a chance to win, but you tell yourself, "I can't win, I've never won before, I'm not good enough." Well, the likely result is that you won't win! Or you keep thinking *I can't get better, the doctors told me my back pain will never go away*. You wake up fearful to start the day because you believe the pain will always be there. These are all limiting, fear-based scenarios—your limiting beliefs.

Instead of imagining your fears, focus on what you want. Visualize your goals and the outcomes you want to achieve, visualize yourself achieving your goals. Visualization is mental practice. When you visualize your desired outcomes, you begin to see the possibility of achieving them.

Visualization is an active state of imagination training or reprogramming for your mind. You guide the breath and mind in a specific direction for a desired result, such as a positive change in mindset, feeling, or bodily sensation. You can use visualization as a tool to prepare your physical, mental, and emotional state for high performance by actively imagining your goals. Yes, it can be hard at first, and it takes work. But over time, you will perform better in those imagined and real situations.

Visualization for sport performance has been around since the 1970s. And many, if not all, elite athletes today use this technique, including golfing great Tiger Woods who has been using it since he was a teenager. These athletes use images in their heads to see their performance and practice it in their heads before the actual event. They engage all their senses in their mental rehearsal to make it more vivid and real. Studies have shown that visualization can increase golf performance by improving coordination and concentration. It also helps with relaxation and reducing fear and anxiety.

The legendary golfer Jack Nicklaus said, "I never hit a shot, not even in practice, without having a very sharp in-focus picture of it in my head. It's like a colour movie. First, I 'see' where I want the ball to finish, nice and white and sitting high on the bright green grass. Then the scene quickly changes, and I 'see' the ball going there: its path, trajectory, and shape, even its behaviour on landing. Then there's sort of a fade-out, the next scene shows me making the kind of swing that will turn the previous images into reality." Jack Nicklaus was one of the first golfers to popularize visualization and is considered to be the greatest golfer of all time.

Research tells us that visualization works because the neurons in your brain (these are the brain cells that transmit information) can't tell the difference between an imagined and real-life action. When you visualize an act, the brain sends a message to your neurons to perform the movement. This creates a new neural pathway, which are clusters of cells in your brain that work together to create memories or learned behaviors. This then trains your body to act in a way consistent to what you imagined. This happens without you actually performing the physical activity, yet it achieves a similar result. Pretty amazing, right? Remember Tammy's story of how visualization helped her win her first provincial golf championship? This stuff works!

Try this quick exercise to experience the power of visualization. It is from the Feldenkrais Method, which is a system of movement education created by Dr. Moshe Feldenkrais (1904-1984), which emphasises self-awareness in sensing, moving, feeling and thinking for integration of mind and body.

Step 1

- Stand up straight in a good solid stance, feet shoulder width apart and firmly planted on the floor or ground.

- Lift your right arm up straight in front of you, fingers pointing. Then turn around to the right with your upper body as far back as you can until you can't turn any further and notice where your fingers are pointing, either to a spot on a wall or landmark of some kind.

- Lock that point into your memory. Get a vivid, digital picture of what you see.

- Now turn around and come back to centre and lower your arm.

Step 2
- While you are standing there, close your eyes and just imagine you are lifting that right arm and turning your upper body around to the right as far as you can. In your mind, you see your fingers pointing at that initial endpoint when you physically turned and now visualize yourself turning your upper body even further, another foot or two past that end point. There's no strain, no effort, no pain. You're just able to turn further.
- Lock a new mental picture in your head of where your fingers are now pointing, noticing how much further past it is from where they pointed before. Make the image very clear and vivid, see it in colour, visualize it as clearly as you can.
- Now imagine bringing your arm back to centre and lowering it down to your side.
- You can open your eyes.

Step3
- Now you are going to physically do the same motion you did in Step 1. Raise your right arm

up one more time and turn your upper body around to the right as far as you can.

- See how far you can go and notice where your fingers are pointing.

Find Your Focus

One of the best ways to get focused in the moment is to train your mind to pay attention to only one thing. This can be accomplished through the practice of meditation, which has been around for centuries, going back to 1500 BC. Meditation is used to train attention and awareness and achieve a clear mind and calm state. It has many health benefits, such as reducing stress and pain, and increasing inner peace and well-being.

Meditation is a practice we've both incorporated into our lives over the past ten years, and we practice it daily. It's had a huge, positive impact on our mental and physical well-being, and it's helped improve our golf.

During a round of golf, you're likely to face challenges that can throw you off your game plan and make you react impulsively, in a negative way. This results in mental mistakes that often cost you strokes. But with regular meditation you can remain mindful and in the moment. You'll learn to keep your thoughts separate from your emotions, allowing you to make more positive and effective decisions.

Through a type of meditation called mindfulness meditation, you can learn how to block out distractions and sounds during your round of golf that disrupt your thoughts. You'll have better self-control and a more positive mindset. You'll learn how to stay calm between shots and focused during your shot. During competition, it will help you stay patient to outlast your opponent. You won't decide to make that risky shot right after you hit a bad one. Just think—no more double bogeys!

Over time, these positive experiences compound and will increase your confidence in your game. Your score will improve, and you'll have more fun.

Meditation is not only beneficial for improving golf performance, research shows it has many other health benefits as well.

- It improves your sleep.
- It lessens anxiety.
- It lessens tension.
- It increases happiness.

We've created a short meditation for you to experience. Please go to our YouTube channel, Hole In One Success, and give it a try. You can find many other examples of meditations on YouTube as well. Try a few and see which ones work best for you. We find mindfulness meditation works best for us, ten to twenty minutes every morning. The key is to practice it regularly, so it becomes a habit. You can listen to guided or non-guided meditations, whatever suits your tastes. We do both.

Practicing the techniques in this chapter will help you strengthen that mind-body connection for playing better golf. If you build them into your day and make them a habit, you'll have more focus and concentration, fewer aches and pains, and you'll swing the club better. The benefits are amazing!

Chapter 6:

Block Therapy Fore Golf

This chapter will fully introduce you to the phenomenal new self-care bodywork practice that can move you from pain and poor mobility to peak performance in your golf game—and your life.

This technique is called Block Therapy, founded by Deanna Hansen, an athletic therapist from Winnipeg, Manitoba, Canada. Block Therapy is a self-care bodywork technique that helps release compressed fascia and bring space and life back to your cells. It is a therapy, exercise, and meditation all in one modality.

Let's look at a scenario to help explain. One of our students, Jim, was getting ready for his first game of the golf season. He did some light stretching then off he went to the first tee. *Swack!* Ouch! He felt a painful tweak in lower left side of his back. Does this sound familiar? Many of us think we've stretched enough and warmed up our muscles when we really haven't. The fascia surrounding the muscles have become glued together over time due to compression from poor posture, aging, stress, and even gravity. The only thing that will fully release this seal is sustained pressure in one area for at least three minutes or more while doing diaphragmatic breathing.

Block Therapy does this. The technique uses this wooden tool called the "block buddy." Yes, this is the piece of magic wood that saved Barry's back! The block buddy is a specially crafted piece of cedar or bamboo shaped to fit all contours of the body. The person lays on this tool in certain positions while breathing using their diaphragm. The block applies pressure on an area of your body that has compression or adhesions. Through diaphragmatic breathing, it allows you to release that compressed tissue, bringing increased blood and oxygen flow to the area. With gravity and body weight, the block buddy can sink deeply into the tissue all the way to the bone. This pressure brings increased blood and oxygen into the area warming the connective tissue and "melting" the powerful seal between the layers of unhealthy restrictions. Combined with diaphragmatic breathing and postural awareness training, this increases mobility, brings relief from chronic pain and creates a whole new level of body awareness at a deeper level.

The benefits of block therapy are countless, many of them a listed below:

- Releases chronic pain.
- Improves mobility, flexibility and strength.

- Increases energy levels.
- Improves posture.
- Releases stress.
- Improves focus and concentration.
- Improves mindset.
- Improves circulation .
- Improves skin tone and body shape.
- Improves digestion and elimination.
- Facilitates weight loss.
- Releases negative emotions.

We both have experienced all of these benefits since incorporating Block Therapy into our lives. Not only will it bring health back to your body, it will bring better movement and energy back to your golf game.

The key areas of your body that require good mobility for your golf game are your hips, back, shoulders, core, knees, and feet. These areas are targeted through the Block Therapy technique to release compressed tissue, allowing you to swing more freely and without pain.

The act of incorporating conscious diaphragmatic breathing and proper posture with fascia decompression is what makes this practice different from anything else. Besides having a positive impact on your health as you age, it has a clear and profound impact on the mind-body connection. As you release compressed fascia, you are also releasing years of pent-up tension, toxins, and negative emotions from your body, freeing yourself to move better, feel better, and play better golf.

One of our students, Judy, who's in her late fifties, had severe pain in her left hip when she golfed. Every time she swung the club, there was jarring pain at the end of the swing. She knew when it was coming on, and she would always flinch at the end of her swing. Over time, this caused her to not rotate her hips fully all the way through because she was anticipating the pain. She would rotate only three quarters of the way through. Her arms would either wrap around or stay out to the right. Other parts of her body were compensating for the immobility in her hip. The resulting golf shot was usually not good.

We got her started on a Block Therapy program that addressed her specific mobility issues. Once she was shown the technique, she was able to do the therapy herself at home. She does it for at least fifteen minutes a day. This technique released all the compressed fascia in her hip, which was the primary pain site. But she also worked in the ribcage, core area, and her legs, which were cause sites for the pain. The fascia released over time and the pain completely disappeared. At sixty years old, she can now swing fully through the ball and has gained 20 yards off the tee!

Get on the block! That's a common phrase said by everyone as they move through their Block Therapy journey with us. Anytime we get pain of any sort, that's what we do, we get on the block. Block Therapy really is the missing link for a healthy body and a better golf game!

Block Fore Golf Program

In partnership with the founder of Block Therapy, Deanna Hansen, we created an online Block Fore Golf program several years ago designed specifically for golfers. It addresses the areas of your body that are specific to the golf swing and will help improve your mobility, flexibility, and swing motion. We are presenting some of the key Block Fore Golf positions below so that you can better understand how this will help your golf game and improve your health. You would basically be lying over the block buddy with your body and following a prescribed technique.

Belly: We always start with the belly position so that you can heat up your core and get the diaphragm working more efficiently. This also helps strengthen the core. Increased blood and oxygen to this area ensures the organs and muscles are functioning properly and will reduce any compression. This area is actually a cause site for back pain. Did you know about 70 percent of your immune system is in your abdominal cavity?

Diaphragm and ribs: Working these areas helps you to open the thoracic area (the rib cage) to ensure you can turn better in the golf swing. The turn in a golf swing is from the upper body, not the lower back.

Hip flexors: The hip flexors are a key muscle for moving your hips and legs. They become shortened and tight from too much sitting and cause pain in the lower back. You want to release the compression in this area. This helps with the hip turn and relieves back pain as now the lower back doesn't have to compensate.

<u>Shoulders and pectorals</u>: In the upper body, you want to release compressed fascia around the shoulders, pecs, and sternum. This area gets very tight from shallow upper chest breathing, poor posture, and sitting hunched over a desk or computer all day. Freeing up the fascia in this area will increase your range of motion in your shoulder so that you can easily make full shoulder turns during the golf swing.

<u>Legs</u>: Moving into the leg area, you will work on the adductors, quadriceps, hamstrings, calves and feet. This will improve circulation in the legs and feet, which are the foundation for the golf swing. It will aid the alignment of your legs and feet with your pelvis and facilitate proper hip turn. You want to ensure that your foundation is strong with no restrictions.

There are a few circumstances where Block Therapy may not be recommended—women who are pregnant, people with steel rods in their back, and those with large surgical mesh in their bodies. We always discuss these situations with our students ahead of time to ensure they are safe.

There is an occurrence in Block Therapy called a "healing crisis". This can happen when you block any area of the body and it begins to move back into its proper postural alignment. Often this occurs when blocking the rib cage. Over time as your posture worsens, your rib cage collapses into your core and moves out of its natural alignment.

The ribs then literally become "glued" out of place because of the compressed fascia. When blocking, the rib releases due to the melting process. It becomes unglued from the others and begins to move back into its proper alignment. This can cause pain for some people for a short period. The usual response is to ice the area. However, when you go through the Block Therapy program, we teach that the better response is to apply heat, not ice, to the area. Icing cools the tissue, and the natural healing process of the body is slowed down. Heat warms the area and aids the healing process. Once the pain dissipates you will feel *so* much better. Your body is moving itself back into proper alignment.

Other instances of a healing crisis could be rashes appearing on your body, excess mucus draining from your nose, or you could have emotional releases as well. These are all natural reactions, as your body is getting rid of toxins and bringing fresh blood and oxygen into your cells to make them healthier.

Barry's Story

I remember this one winter when we flew to Maui for a vacation, I had been blocking for about four months. When we landed, my back and ribs were a bit stiff, which I chalked up to sitting in a cramped airplane seat for six hours. When I grabbed my travel golf bag off the airport luggage carrousel, I felt a slight twinge in my thoracic area, but thought nothing of it. The next day we drove to a local flea market to get some fresh produce and see what other treasures we might find. I parked the van, opened the door, and turned my upper body to get out of the driver's seat. All of a sudden, excruciating pain surged through the left side of my ribs. I could not move! I yelled out in pain, which is pretty rare for me, as I have quite a high pain tolerance. Tammy came running around from the passenger side to see what was wrong. It was quite painful and I felt I should go to the hospital, it was that bad!

Tammy drove me to a local hospital nearby and tests were done, but nothing serious was found, just seemed to be some rib muscle inflammation. The doctor gave me pain killers, and we headed back to our villa. It then became apparent to me that this was likely a rib release. I had been blocking my ribs quite a bit before we left for vacation. I guess when I picked up that travel golf bag, it tweaked enough to release the rib from its incorrect position, and thus the pain the next day. But ... I had my block buddy with me (we never travel without them), and I knew exactly what to do. I gently blocked around the area of the rib release, and I applied heat between my blocking sessions. Never ice! After a day, the pain dissipated, and I felt better than ever! My thoracic area felt more open, and I could turn more freely. Golf swing—no problem! A healing crisis, if you have one, always leaves you feeling so much better once it's over.

This unique practice has been a life saver for us; it's given us back our health and our golf as we move into the second half of our lives. And this is something you can do for yourself as well. You can learn more about our Block Fore Golf program through our website link at the end of this book.

Chapter 7:

Swing into Action

Now is the time to take what you've learned in this book and put it into action. As we discussed in Chapter 4, you need to set goals and then take action for change to occur. We talked about chunking things down and making a small list of daily actions to keep it manageable. Now you need to schedule those actions.

What Gets Scheduled Gets Done

Schedule your actions somewhere they can be easily accessed, so you won't forget about them. If you are tech-savvy, there are a lot of great online calendars. Your smart phone has a calendar. Google has a calendar. Pick whatever one meets your needs, as long as you can schedule in the actions with a time and date. If you are old school, use a paper calendar or one of those organizers with extra room to write the actions and other related information, such as your goals. Photocopy it and paste on your fridge. The important thing here is to schedule the action. What gets scheduled gets done!

Let's talk about commitment. What is your level of commitment? Are you kind of committed? 90 percent committed? That won't work. Think about it. What happens in your golf swing if you are "kind of" committed to the swing? The golf shot usually doesn't work out, right? You need to be 100 percent committed to taking action or success will be harder to achieve, or you won't achieve it at all. You've come this far though, so that tells us you are committed and you will follow through.

Let's go back to the rule of five we discussed in Chapter 4. Schedule five things in your calendar you know you can accomplish every day. This could be five small tasks that contribute to one larger goal. For example, if you committed to work out every day for thirty minutes, your actions could be broken down into ten minutes of walking in the morning, a ten-minute stretch over lunch, or ten minutes of diaphragmatic breathing and posture reset at night. They can be simple things that don't overwhelm you but still allow you to achieve your results. Remember, nothing will change until you do, it starts with you taking action.

Check in with Yourself

Okay, you're really swinging into action! You're moving toward playing your best golf over fifty and enjoying the back nine to the fullest. No bogeys, no double bogeys, only pars or better. What a great feeling! And it's not just on the golf course, it's off the golf course as well. Your calendar is filled with your actions. Awesome! But wouldn't it be great to have someone or something to help you stay on track? This is where an accountability partner comes in.

Accountability partners help you stay positively focused on your goals and successes, rather than on your mistakes and shortcomings. An accountability partner will check in with you every day, if you want, to see if you are following through on your action plan. Are you sticking with your golf lessons? Are you doing your fitness and mobility program? They will check in to see how you are doing, how you are feeling about things, and whether you need to make any changes. They may challenge you to complete an action that you've been putting off. The key thing is they will help you stay positive even when there are shortcomings, challenges, and failures (which are really steps to success). So you can see why it's very worthwhile to get an accountability partner. It could be your spouse, a coach, a friend, or a sibling. Anyone, as long as you and this person are both committed to connecting on a regular basis. You can have more than one accountability partner if you like, depending on the areas you need support in. One partner could be for the fitness, another could be for golf technique. Whatever works best for you.

The important thing to remember here is that accountability is key to make sure things happen. It's easy to make excuses and not take action when no one is checking in to see if you have followed through. With an accountability partner, there is no blaming, no shaming, no judgment or guilt trips, just positive support to help you take action toward your goals.

We've both had several accountability partners over the past few years, and they have propelled us along to great lengths. We probably wouldn't have written this book if it weren't for the help of our accountability partners!

Create New Habits

You've completed a lot of great work if you've followed through on the exercises in this book. The intent is for all that hard work to lead you to the best back nine of your life. All the tools and techniques and information have set you up for developing new positive habits.

What are habits? Habits are thoughts about things that over time become a reality if you do them repeatedly. As you've discovered in this book, some habits can serve you poorly. They are habits developed over your lifetime that are stopping you from being your best. Now is the time for you to break those bad habits and create better ones.

To create a new habit, research shows that you must continually practice the new action, thought, feeling, or technique for at least twenty-one to thirty days, so your brain can rewire itself and make the habit automatic. That's why it's so important to stick to your golf lesson plan and do the drills as often as you can. Repeat, repeat, repeat. Train your body to move in a new way, make it a habit. There is an old quote from a Latin proverb that says,

"Repetition is the mother of all learning." The more we repeat something, the better we become at it.

One way to create a new habit is to try a twenty-one-day challenge in an area where you want to make a positive change. This could be something you discuss with your coach. It could be a prescribed lesson and practice challenge where you are at the range or golf course every day. It could be an online challenge where you listen to live teachings and have homework each night. It could be something you agreed to with your accountability partner, who will check in with you every day. There are many ways to approach it, but the concept here is to do something for at least twenty-one days to make it a habit. Things you may have found difficult in the past, like committing to exercise every day, are good challenges, because after twenty-one days you have a much better chance of making it a permanent behavior.

Tammy's Story

In my first twenty-one-day challenge with Block Therapy, I lost eight pounds, got rid of my hip and shoulder pain, and learned how to breathe properly. I created a habit to block every day for at least fifteen minutes. Now it has become a daily habit, and on many days, I end up blocking even longer. It's enough to make a big difference in how I feel every day. I was so excited about my results from this challenge that I trained in the Block Therapy technique, and I'm now certified to teach it to others. It has changed my life. Creating a new habit can change yours as well.

Chapter 8:

Your Scorecard for Success

Many of you keep score when you play golf so you know how many shots you've hit. But you should also keep score on your journey to better golf after fifty so you know whether you are making progress toward your goals. Monitoring and tracking your progress will keep you motivated. It will help reinforce the actions you are taking to get your results, creating more positive habits.

One way to track you progress is to simply keep a golf journal to record what's working well and where you need improvement. After each round of golf or practice session, take a few minutes to reflect on your performance. Ask yourself what you did well, what you could have done better, and what you need to improve on for next time. Jot down some notes on this and also how you felt during the round or practice session. Use this information to help you plan your next course of action and set some new goals.

You can also keep statistics on each round of golf you play. This will help you assess specifically where you're improving in your game, and what areas you need to spend more time on.

Possible statistics to include are:

- Number of strokes you take for each hole, including any penalties, to determine how close to par you are.
- Percentage of fairways you hit each round (does not include par 3s). You should strive for at least 50 percent or better.
- Percentage of greens hit in regulation (within the expected number of shots). For a par 4 it's two, for a par 5 it's three. If you're a bogey golfer, 20-25 percent is average. As you move up to scratch player, 50-60 percent is what you want to strive for.
- Number of putts per round. Less than thirty-six is ideal. The lower, the better.
- Number of sand saves, which is holing out in two strokes once you land in a greenside bunker.
- Number of up and downs, which is the consistency with which you hole out in two shots after you miss the green with your approach shot (and are not in the bunker).

By no means do you have to keep all these stats, but those who do are more focused on the areas they need to improve upon. Keeping track of your stats helps you practice more effectively. There are many apps available for keeping these stats.

Monitoring progress and keeping score for success will give you a great sense of accomplishment. Seeing where you're at and how far you've come can be very motivating to keep you moving toward your goals. The act of writing things down and then reviewing what you've accomplished allows it sink into your subconscious and reinforce your actions. Review your notes regularly. Then share your progress with others. This will make you feel good about yourself and give you confidence.

Feedback is Your Friend

Many people don't like receiving feedback because they take it as criticism, but using feedback can make the difference between success and failure. There are many sources of feedback. It could come from your playing partners or coach. It can come from the environment or from your own performance. Often golfers criticize themselves on the course for their poor shots or poor performance instead of looking at these as opportunities for feedback.

Maybe you hit a slice off the first tee. That's feedback telling you something about your swing path and clubface alignment. But many wouldn't think of this as feedback, they'd see it as just a bad swing.

When you have that 4-foot putt and miss it on the low side, consistently, that's feedback you are either aiming too low or closing your putter face. Now that you have this feedback, you can re-adjust your putting alignment and make corrections.

If you get a sore back when you play, or you can't turn your hips through the ball, that's feedback your body has problems in those areas that need to be addressed. You need to pay attention to this feedback so you can make the necessary changes and adjustments to get yourself back on track.

Look for patterns in your feedback, what are they telling you? Patterns are important as they can tell you things you wouldn't necessarily notice in a one-time occurrence. Pay attention.

Feedback can be both positive and negative, so don't discount anything. Both kinds are useful and will move you forward. Watch for different kinds of feedback while you play, listen to what other people say about your game and use it to your advantage. Don't discard it as just criticism. Every bit of feedback is useful in some way or another.

Tammy's Story

I remember when I first joined a private club. I was a newbie but quickly found a small group of golfing friends that I played with quite often, and we had a lot of fun. Little did I know that, behind my back, they were constantly complaining about my slow play to each other. One day, one of my playing partners called me aside after a round and finally told me that I had a reputation at the club for slow play. At first, I was shocked and hurt. I didn't believe her. Me? Slow? No way! And why had she waited so long to say anything to me? I felt betrayed by all of them. I was upset for days but that wasn't helping the situation. So then I decided to reflect on my golf rounds. Was I a slow player? Hmm . . . maybe. The next time I played I paid close attention to my pace of play compared to my playing partners. Wow! What an eyeopener! I was like a sloth compared to the others. Why hadn't I seen that before? I was so wrapped up in my own little routine I didn't realize how slow I was. I learned a lot from that feedback and found a way to speed up my play without having to sacrifice my routine. I also thanked my friend for having the guts to give me the feedback on my slow play. It changed how I play the game and has been very helpful as I moved into competitions with pace of play policies. It also just makes the game more fun for everyone.

Persistence Pays Off

You've created your vision, your goals, and action plans, and have implemented the solutions we provided. Stay motivated by practicing persistence. Don't give up. Look for those small wins that will help keep you moving forward. Along the way, there will be some setbacks. That's to be expected. As we said at the beginning, golf is not a game of perfect. Setbacks are a natural part of the process. When faced with setbacks, just step back for a minute and assess what really happened. Don't react in the moment. Breathe. Think it through rationally then come up with a few options to move forward. Weigh the pros and cons and pick the best option. Then just move forward.

If you follow these steps and take action, you'll achieve your goals. And then celebrate your successes. Shout it out! Tell your family and friends. You deserve recognition for the positive changes you made. Feel good about yourself, your game and your health. You've earned it. You did the work, and it paid off. Think back on how far you've come. The journey onward will be so much fun. You have your plan; you know what to do.

Chapter 9:

Your Best Back Nine Ever

Wow! What a journey it's been! You've come so far since you turned that first page of this book. You've discovered more about yourself and why you golf, and what drives you to that passion. You looked at where you are now and where you want to be. You know more about your golf habits. You know your swing faults, the mobility issues that are holding you back, and your mindset patterns. And you've been able to take all of that and come up with a vision for what you want and set goals and build an action plan around that. That is huge!

Next you learned about the golf swing and some of the common swing faults and fixes most golfers have after fifty. And you were given some great drills to do to get you on your way to improving.

Then you read about techniques around the mind-body connection. You learned how you can use your breathing and posture and dynamic mobility techniques to help improve your overall health and swing the club with more ease. You now know more about the new self-care fascia release technique called Block Therapy, which will alleviate your chronic pain and help get your body in the proper swing position for golf. And then we gave you some tips and tools for helping you pull it all together so you can swing into action and start playing your best golf today and every day.

Lastly, we talked about keeping score for success so you can monitor your progress, know where you're at, and feel good about the results you've achieved. We talked about how to use feedback to your advantage and how to stay motivated to succeed. And we also discussed the importance of sharing with others so they can celebrate your successes with you.

These simple tools will have a big impact on your game and your life when you put them into practice. They will set you on a clear path to success.

Let's Carry On

So how are you feeling right now? You've engaged in an amazing journey. The way to success is to follow through with your plan. Believe in yourself and your abilities to be and do your best. Keep up with your daily commitments, record your progress, and set new goals once you've reached the first ones.

You want this to last, right? You want to play and feel your best for as long as you can. This journey is about more than just golf; it's really about your journey on the back nine of life. How do you want it to play out? Do you want pars and birdies? Or maybe you want a hole-in-one! It's all there waiting for you. All you have to do is say yes to yourself. You have likely spent the first half of your life caring for others, addressing other people's needs instead of yours. Now is the time to focus on yourself and your needs. Do the things you're passionate about. Go for it. Don't have second thoughts. Keep moving forward on your journey and have your best back nine ever!

Join Our Community

As you embark upon your back nine, we are here to support you. We have a vibrant and engaged Facebook community of like-minded golfers called "Play Your Best Golf Today." In this community you can ask questions, seek support and guidance, leave comments, and give advice and support to others. We're in there almost every day to answer questions and provide video tips and techniques to help you play your best golf and improve your health. You can even post a swing video of yourself and we will take a look at it and give you some tips and feedback.

It's quite a unique and participatory community that will connect you with other like-minded golfers. The more you engage and ask questions, the more you will get out of it. The key is to keep learning. You will meet fellow golfers from all over the world with similar issues, concerns, and stories to your own. We can learn from each other and get better together.

If you would like to join us on our journey, please reach out to us through our website at www.holeinone-success.com. We would love to work with you. We will personally take you through all the steps we've laid out in this book and guide you every step of the way. We'll help you make the back nine the best nine of your life.

To your success, on and off the course,

Tammy and Barry

About the Authors

Tammy and Barry Gibson are founders of Hole In One Success and golf performance coaches who specialize in helping middle-aged golfers struggling with back pain, poor mobility, and other related health issues to play the best golf of their lives. Their 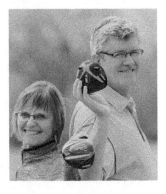 unique approach combines golf instruction, mobility, and mindset into one simple to use system. Tammy is a certified Block Therapy instructor and Fascial Fitness trainer, as well as a Canfield Success Principles trainer. Barry is a PGA of Canada golf professional and top teaching pro with more than thirty years of experience, having coached his wife, Tammy, to five provincial amateur golf championships and over ten national championship appearances. Both are Titleist Performance Institute (TPI) certified for functional movement assessment for the golf swing. Together they have worked with hundreds of golfers to take strokes off their game and improve their health. Tammy and Barry live in Winnipeg, Canada. They can be reached at www.holeinonesuccess.com

A free ebook edition is available with the purchase of this book.

To claim your free ebook edition:

1. Visit MorganJamesBOGO.com
2. Sign your name CLEARLY in the space
3. Complete the form and submit a photo of the entire copyright page
4. You or your friend can download the ebook to your preferred device

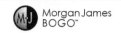

A **FREE** ebook edition is available for you or a friend with the purchase of this print book.

CLEARLY SIGN YOUR NAME ABOVE

Instructions to claim your free ebook edition:
1. Visit MorganJamesBOGO.com
2. Sign your name CLEARLY in the space above
3. Complete the form and submit a photo of this entire page
4. You or your friend can download the ebook to your preferred device

Print & Digital Together Forever.

Snap a photo

Free ebook

Read anywhere

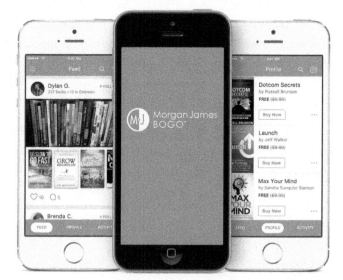

Printed in the USA
CPSIA information can be obtained
at www.ICGtesting.com
JSHW081707170624
64967JS00004B/197

9 781631 954320